Communications
in Computer and Information Science   **665**

Commenced Publication in 2007
Founding and Former Series Editors:
Alfredo Cuzzocrea, Xiaoyong Du, Orhun Kara, Ting Liu, Dominik Ślęzak,
and Xiaokang Yang

More information about this series at http://www.springer.com/series/7899

Habib M. Fardoun · Victor M.R. Penichet
Daniyal M. Alghazzawi · M. Elena De la Guia (Eds.)

ICTs for Improving Patients Rehabilitation Research Techniques

Third International Workshop, REHAB 2015
Lisbon, Portugal, October 1–2, 2015
Revised Selected Papers

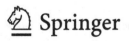 Springer

Editors
Habib M. Fardoun
King Abdulaziz University
Jeddah
Saudi Arabia

Victor M.R. Penichet 🆔
University of Castilla-La Mancha
Albacete
Spain

Daniyal M. Alghazzawi
King Abdulaziz University
Jeddah
Saudi Arabia

M. Elena De la Guia 🆔
University of Castilla-La Mancha
Albacete
Spain

ISSN 1865-0929   ISSN 1865-0937 (electronic)
Communications in Computer and Information Science
ISBN 978-3-319-69693-5   ISBN 978-3-319-69694-2 (eBook)
https://doi.org/10.1007/978-3-319-69694-2

Library of Congress Control Number: 2017957566

Printed on acid-free paper

This Springer imprint is published by Springer Nature
The registered company is Springer International Publishing AG
The registered company address is: Gewerbestrasse 11, 6330 Cham, Switzerland

Preface

During the last few years, there has been increasing interest in the application of virtual reality and information and communication technologies (ICTs) in the field of rehabilitation, with clinical results that prove their effectiveness.

New technologies such as Kinect, virtual reality, sensors, augmented reality, eye tracking, 3D printers, etc. allow us to develop innovative solutions for assistance, prevention, and rehabilitation in patients. In this way, the new technologies can help patients to function more easily in their everyday lives and can also make it easier for a caregiver care them.

The main focus of this book titled *New Technologies to improve Patient Rehabilitation* has been to explore how technology can contribute toward smarter and effective rehabilitation methods. Contained herein are 15 chapters:

Chapter 1 presents a conceptual framework to encourage the research community to develop more comprehensive and adaptive ICT solutions for prevention and rehabilitation of chronic conditions in the daily life of the aging population and beyond health facilities. Chapter 2 investigates and presents a virtual system for balance control assessment that is used to implement a virtual task for balance tracking in real time at home. Chapter 3 explores how gaze tracking (GT) can provide more accurate and direct indicators about the cognitive processes in rehabilitation. Chapter 4 investigates the design and manufacture of medical devices, such as lower limb prosthesis, integrating low-cost industrial technologies. In particular, it focuses attention on the custom-fit component of a lower limb prosthesis, i.e., the socket, that is the interface with the residual limb. Chapter 5 investigates an auditory feedback-based system for treating autism spectrum disorder. The system for real-time gesture tracking is presented, used in active well-being self-assessment activities and in particular applied to medical coaching and music therapy. Chapter 6 presents a balance measurement software based on Kinect2 sensor, which is evaluated by comparison with the Wii balance board in a numerical analysis level, and further improved according to the consideration of BFP (body fat percentage) values of the user. Chapter 7 presents a study testing the efficacy of an alternative mHealth approach using tablets and serious games to stimulate cognitive functions in recovering addicts. In Chapter 8, a balance measurement software based on Kinect2 sensor is evaluated and compared with the gold standard balance measure platform intuitively. The software analysis uses the tracked body data from the user via the Kinect2 sensor and gets the user's center of mass (CoM) and motion route on a plane. Chapter 9 presents a model based on games to improve auditory verbal therapy, which is carried out with deaf children who have benefited from a cochlear implant. In Chapter 10 the author presents how the virtual reality can support a hyperbaric oxygen therapy. In Chapter 11, the authors have devised a system based on the combined use of low-cost virtual reality visors, like Google Cardboard, and ad hoc developed games for smartphones to improve amblyopia. Chapter 12 provides a summary of previous studies that incorporated computer games for CP rehabilitation.

Moreover, a comprehensive game-based rehabilitation framework is presented to enable CP children to actively participate in upper-limb physical exercises. Chapter 13 reports a study in which the authors tested the relation between neuropsychological functions and abstinence after an alcohol rehabilitation treatment. Chapter 14 analyzes how the interaction process of editing exercises in a virtual rehabilitation environment is affected when using Web applications and devices such as Microsoft Kinect. Chapter 15 presents the experiment and design of a system for rhythmic rehabilitation based on a stationary bike augmented in an audio reality.

Finally, we would like to thank all authors for the valuable contributions presented, all the organizers (King Abdulaziz University and ISE Research group UCLM) and collaborators (COPELABS, Lusophone University, Lisbon, Portugal), together with the reviewers (members of the Program Committee) for helping us by contributing to a high-quality book on the topics of rehabilitation.

September 2017

Habib M. Fardoun
Victor M.R. Penichet
Daniyal M. Alghazzawi
M. Elena De la Guia

Organization

King Abdulaziz University and ISE Research group (UCLM).

Chairs and Program Co-chairs

Habib M. Fardoun   King Abdulaziz University, Saudi Arabia
Victor M.R. Penichet   University of Castilla-La Mancha, Spain
Daniyal M. Alghazzawi   King Abdulaziz University, Saudi Arabia
M. Elena De la Guia   University of Castilla-La Mancha, Spain

Organizing Committee

Pedro Gamito   COPELABS, Lusophone University, Portugal
Sergio Albiol Pérez   University of Zaragoza, Spain

Technical Coordination

Juan Enrique Garrido   University of Castilla-La Mancha, Spain

Program Committee

Belinda Lange   Institute for Creative Technologies, University of Southern
                          California, USA
Willem-Paul Brinkman   Delft University of Technology, The Netherlands
Mariano Luis Alcañiz   Instituto Interuniversitario de Investigación en
                          Bioingeniería, Spain
Beatriz Rey   Universidad Politécnica de Valencia, Spain
Imre Cikajlo   Univerzitetni rehabilitacijski inštitut Republike Slovenije,
                          Slovenia
Roberto Lloréns   Instituto Interuniversitario de Investigación en
                          Bioingeniería, Spain
José Antonio Gil   Universidad Politécnica de Valencia, Spain
Mónica Cameirão   University of Madeira, Portugal
Sergi Bermudez   University of Madeira, Portugal
Emily Keshner   Temple University, USA
Hermenegildo Gil   Universidad Politécnica de Valencia, Spain
Kjartan Halvorsen   Uppsala University, Sweden
Thalmann Daniel   University of Paul Sabatier, France
Rosa Maria E. Moreira   Universidade do Estado do Rio de Janeiro, Brazil

Contents

Towards Pervasive Predictive Analytics in Interactive Prevention
and Rehabilitation for Older People 1
    Maria Claudia Buzzi, Marina Buzzi, and Amaury Trujillo

A Virtual System for Balance Control Assessment at Home 12
    Matteo Spezialetti, Daniela Iacoviello, Andrea Petracca,
    and Giuseppe Placidi

Assessment of Attentional and Mnesic Processes Through Gaze Tracking
Analysis: Inferences from Comparative Search Tasks Embedded
in VR Serious Games 26
    Pedro J. Rosa, Diogo Morais, Jorge Oliveira, Pedro Gamito,
    Olivia Smyth, and Matthew Pavlovic

Pressure Data and Multi-material Approach to Design Prosthesis 35
    Claudio Comotti, Daniele Regazzoni, Caterina Rizzi, and Andrea Vitali

An Auditory Feedback Based System for Treating Autism
Spectrum Disorder 46
    Massimo Magrini, Andrea Carboni, Ovidio Salvetti, and Olivia Curzio

Using Wii Balance Board to Evaluate Software Based on Kinect2 59
    Zhihan Lv, Vicente Penades, Sonia Blasco, Javier Chirivella,
    and Pablo Gagliardo

Cognitive Improvement via mHealth for Patients Recovering
from Substance Use Disorder 69
    B. Rosa, J. Oliveira, P. Gamito, P. Lopes, D. Morais, R. Brito,
    C. Caçoête, A. Leandro, T. Almeida, and H. Oliveira

Intuitively Evaluating Balance Measurement Software Using Kinect2 83
    Zhihan Lv, Vicente Penades, Sonia Blasco, Javier Chirivella,
    and Pablo Gagliardo

Model for Design of Serious Game for Rehabilitation in Children
with Cochlear Implant 94
    Sandra Cano, Victor Peñeñory, César Collazos, Habib M. Fardoun,
    and Daniyal M. Alghazzawi

Hyperbaric Oxygen Chamber Users May Obtain Immersive Enjoyment
by Virtual Reality Glasses 106
    Zhihan Lv

Amblyopia Rehabilitation by Games for Low-Cost Virtual Reality Visors . . .   116
    Silvia Bonfanti and Angelo Gargantini

Interactive Kinect-Based Rehabilitation Framework for Assisting Children
with Upper Limb Cerebral Palsy.   126
    Mohammad I. Daoud, Rami Alazrai, Abdullah Alhusseini, Dima Shihan,
    Ekhlass Alhwayan, Dhiah el Diehn I. Abou-Tair, and Talal Qadoummi

Neuropsychological Predictors of Alcohol Abtinence Following
a Detoxification Program   141
    Bruno Bento, Jorge Oliveira, Fátima Gameiro, Rodrigo Brito,
    Pedro Gamito, Paulo Lopes, Diogo Morais, and Margarida Neto

Virtual Rehabilitation on the Web: Analyzing and Improving Interaction
in Postures Design   150
    Félix Albertos-Marco, José Antonio Fernández Valls,
    Víctor M.R. Penichet, María Dolores Lozano, and José A. Gallud

A Stationary Bike in Augmented Audio Reality. An Investigation
on Soundscapes Influence on Preferred Biking Speed   162
    Justyna Maculewicz and Stefania Serafin

Author Index   179

List of Contributors

Dhiah el Diehn I. Abou-Tair School of Electrical Engineering and Information Technology, German Jordanian University, Amman, Jordan

Rami Alazrai School of Electrical Engineering and Information Technology, German Jordanian University, Amman, Jordan

Félix Albertos-Marco Computer Systems Department, University of Castilla-La Mancha, Albacete, Spain

Daniyal M. Alghazzawi King Abdulaziz University, Jeddah, Saudi Arabia

Abdullah Alhusseini School of Electrical Engineering and Information Technology, German Jordanian University, Amman, Jordan

Ekhlass Alhwayan School of Electrical Engineering and Information Technology, German Jordanian University, Amman, Jordan

T. Almeida Ares do Pinhal Addiction Rehabilitation Association, Lisbon, Portugal

Bruno Bento EPCV/Lusophone University, Campo Grande, 376, Lisbon, Portugal; Casa de Saúde do Telhal, Mem-Martins, Portugal

Sonia Blasco FIVAN, Valencia, Spain

Silvia Bonfanti Università degli Studi di Bergamo, Bergamo, Italy

Rodrigo Brito EPCV/Lusophone University, Campo Grande, 376, Lisbon, Portugal; EPCV and COPELABS/Lusophone University, Campo Grande, 376, Lisbon, Portugal

Maria Claudia Buzzi IIT-CNR, Pisa, Italy

Marina Buzzi IIT-CNR, Pisa, Italy

Sandra Cano LIDIS Group, University of San Buenaventura, Cali, Colombia

Andrea Carboni ISTI – CNR, Pisa, Italy

C. Caçoête Ares do Pinhal Addiction Rehabilitation Association, Lisbon, Portugal

Javier Chirivella FIVAN, Valencia, Spain

César Collazos IDIS Group, University of Cauca, Popayán, Colombia

Claudio Comotti Department of Management, Information and Production Engineering, University of Bergamo, Bergamo, Italy

Olivia Curzio IFC – CNR, Pisa, Italy

Mohammad I. Daoud School of Electrical Engineering and Information Technology, German Jordanian University, Amman, Jordan

Habib M. Fardoun King Abdulaziz University, Jeddah, Saudi Arabia

José Antonio Fernández Valls Computer Science Research Institute (I3A), University of Castilla-La Mancha, Albacete, Spain

Pablo Gagliardo FIVAN, Valencia, Spain

Fátima Gameiro EPCV/Lusophone University, Campo Grande, 376, Lisbon, Portugal; EPCV and COPELABS/Lusophone University, Campo Grande, 376, Lisbon, Portugal

Pedro Gamito ECPV, Universidade Lusófona de Humanidades e Tecnologias, Lisbon, Portugal; School of Psychology and Life Sciences, COPELABS–ULHT, Lisbon, Portugal

José A. Gallud Computer Systems Department, University of Castilla-La Mancha, Albacete, Spain

Angelo Gargantini Università degli Studi di Bergamo, Bergamo, Italy

Daniela Iacoviello Department of Computer, Control and Management Engineering Antonio Ruberti, Sapienza University of Rome, Rome, Italy

A. Leandro Ares do Pinhal Addiction Rehabilitation Association, Lisbon, Portugal

Paulo Lopes EPCV/Lusophone University, Campo Grande, 376, Lisbon, Portugal; EPCV and COPELABS/Lusophone University, Campo Grande, 376, Lisbon, Portugal

María Dolores Lozano Computer Systems Department, University of Castilla-La Mancha, Albacete, Spain

Zhihan Lv FIVAN, Valencia, Spain

Justyna Maculewicz M-LAB, Aalborg University Copenhagen, Copenhagen, Denmark

Massimo Magrini ISTI – CNR, Pisa, Italy

Diogo Morais ECPV, Universidade Lusófona de Humanidades e Tecnologias, Lisbon, Portugal; School of Psychology and Life Sciences, COPELABS–ULHT, Lisbon, Portugal

Margarida Neto Casa de Saúde do Telhal, Mem-Martins, Portugal

Jorge Oliveira ECPV, Universidade Lusófona de Humanidades e Tecnologias, Lisbon, Portugal; School of Psychology and Life Sciences, COPELABS–ULHT, Lisbon, Portugal

H. Oliveira Ares do Pinhal Addiction Rehabilitation Association, Lisbon, Portugal

Matthew Pavlovic University of Michigan, Michigan, USA

Vicente Penades FIVAN, Valencia, Spain

Víctor M.R. Penichet Computer Systems Department, University of Castilla-La Mancha, Albacete, Spain

Andrea Petracca A^2VI_Lab, c/o Department of Life, Health and Environmental Sciences, University of L'Aquila, L'aquila, Italy

Victor Peñeñory LIDIS Group, University of San Buenaventura, Cali, Colombia

Giuseppe Placidi A^2VI_Lab, c/o Department of Life, Health and Environmental Sciences, University of L'Aquila, L'aquila, Italy

Talal Qadoummi School of Electrical Engineering and Information Technology, German Jordanian University, Amman, Jordan

Daniele Regazzoni Department of Management, Information and Production Engineering, University of Bergamo, Bergamo, Italy

Caterina Rizzi Department of Management, Information and Production Engineering, University of Bergamo, Bergamo, Italy

B. Rosa EPCV/Lusophone University, Campo Grande, 376, Lisbon, Portugal; COPELABS/Lusophone University, Campo Grande, 376, Lisbon, Portugal

Pedro J. Rosa ECPV, Universidade Lusófona de Humanidades e Tecnologias, Lisbon, Portugal; School of Psychology and Life Sciences, COPELABS–ULHT, Lisbon, Portugal; Instituto Universitário de Lisboa (ISCTE-IUL), Cis-IUL, Lisbon, Portugal; Centro de Investigação em Psicologia do ISMAT, Portimão, Portugal

Ovidio Salvetti ISTI – CNR, Pisa, Italy

Stefania Serafin M-LAB, Aalborg University Copenhagen, Copenhagen, Denmark

Dima Shihan School of Electrical Engineering and Information Technology, German Jordanian University, Amman, Jordan

Olivia Smyth University of Michigan, Michigan, USA

Matteo Spezialetti A2VI_Lab, c/o Department of Life, Health and Environmental Sciences, University of L'Aquila, L'aquila, Italy

Amaury Trujillo IIT-CNR, Pisa, Italy

Andrea Vitali Department of Management, Information and Production Engineering, University of Bergamo, Bergamo, Italy

Towards Pervasive Predictive Analytics in Interactive Prevention and Rehabilitation for Older People

Maria Claudia Buzzi, Marina Buzzi, and Amaury Trujillo[(✉)]

IIT-CNR, Via Moruzzi 1, Pisa, Italy
{claudia.buzzi,marina.buzzi,
amaury.trujillo}@iit.cnr.it

Abstract. The world population is rapidly aging and becoming a burden to health systems around the world. In this work we present a conceptual framework to encourage the research community to develop more comprehensive and adaptive ICT solutions for prevention and rehabilitation of chronic conditions in the daily life of the aging population and beyond health facilities. We first present an overview of current international standards in human functioning and disability, and how chronic conditions are interconnected in older age. We then describe innovative mobile and sensor technologies, predictive data analysis in healthcare, and game-based prevention and rehabilitation techniques. We then set forth a multidisciplinary approach for the personalized prevention and rehabilitation of chronic conditions using unobtrusive and pervasive sensors, interactive activities, and predictive analytics, which also eases the tasks of health-related researchers, caregivers and providers. Our proposal represents a conceptual basis for future research, in which much remains to be done in terms of standardization of technologies and health terminology, as well as data protection and privacy legislation.

Keywords: Data collection · Telerehabilitation · Computer-assisted therapy

1 Introduction

Rising life expectancy and lower birth rates are the main causes of the world population's aging, especially in the most economically developed countries offering widespread access to healthcare. However, older people (ages 65 and above) are more likely to develop co-morbid conditions that impair their cognitive and physical functioning [1], negatively affecting their Quality of Life (QoL) and increasing the burden on health systems. Due to the complex nature of these chronic conditions, most research studies focus on one or at most two chronic conditions at the same time. Unfortunately, the interconnection and frequent co-occurrence of these conditions makes it difficult to obtain an accurate description of the pathology and treatment of a single condition, especially in older adults. Recent advances in information and communication technology (ICT) allow us to develop innovative solutions for assistance, prevention and rehabilitation used for and by older people, such as sensor technology [2] and virtual reality [3]. In addition, the convergence to connected devices

© Springer International Publishing AG 2017
H.M. Fardoun et al. (Eds.): REHAB 2015, CCIS 665, pp. 1–11, 2017.
https://doi.org/10.1007/978-3-319-69694-2_1

and services via the Internet of Things (IoT), Cloud computing, and Big Data techniques allow us to rapidly collect and analyze enormous volumes of diverse and valuable data like never before. Moreover, it is now possible to use these technologies to develop predictive and adaptive interventions for personalized healthcare.

Therefore, as stated in a previous paper [4], we believe that it is necessary to move forward and combine these advances in ICT to create a more holistic approach for healthy aging in terms of prevention, minimization of negative effects, and rehabilitation of chronic conditions beyond the walls of health facilities. Moreover, we think that the shift of data collection and analysis from health facilities to the daily-life activities of older people (e.g., at home, at the workplace, on the move) will increase their empowerment and reduce the burden on society health costs. In this work, we give a more detailed overview of the motivations, technologies and standards of our proposed conceptual model to attain this goal, which is based on established and internationally validated concepts of human functioning and disability.

2 Health Conditions and Functioning Level in Older Age

The health status of a person is determined by decisive contextual factors inherent to the individual (personal factors), as well as to their socio-economical and physical environments (environmental factors). In particular, contextual factors associated with the increased rate of an ensuing disease (or condition) are defined as risk factors for that condition. These contextual factors can be further classified into modifiable and non-modifiable, according to the individual possibility of change. Nonetheless, sometimes this classification is not straightforward. For instance, some factors that are traditionally considered non-modifiable can be controlled, or as demonstrated by studies in epigenetics their effects can be reduced by environmental changes [5]. Modifiable behavioral determinants are of particular research interest because they can influence the effectiveness of preventive, curative and rehabilitative modes of intervention for healthy aging [6]. For instance, smoking status, physical activity level, body mass index, diet, and alcohol use are lifestyle factors associated with health status in older age [7].

People's health determinants (illustrated in Fig. 1), and consequently health status, change over time; thus, people's functioning level does not remain constant, and they may experience some form of disability in their life. To classify this level of functioning, the World Health Organization (WHO) developed the International Classification of Functioning, Disability and Health (ICF). This standard was born from the need to interlink health information systems in a common and accessible manner, to compare data across systems, disciplines and countries. ICF provides a framework for classification regarding people's body function and structure, what individuals with a health condition can do in a standard environment (level of ability), and what they actually do in their usual environment (level of performance). In ICF, disability and functioning are viewed as outcomes of interactions between health conditions (diseases, disorders and injuries) and contextual factors (personal and environmental).

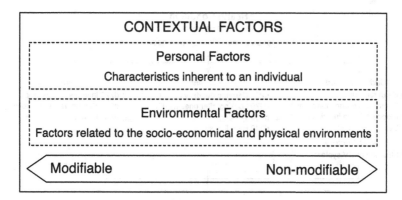

Fig. 1. Health determinants are decisive contextual factors that affect our health

ICF does not classify people but describes their functioning profiles, which are not derived from diagnostic criteria. In this sense, it is complementary to the International Classification of Diseases (ICD), the standard diagnostic tool for epidemiology, health management, and clinical purposes. Both standards help monitor people's health information, in terms of disease and other prevalent conditions, as well as the impact of interventions in the experience of functioning, even when the medical diagnosis remains unchanged. For instance, two people may have the same chronic condition, as described by ICD, but different functioning levels, as described by ICF. Moreover, this functioning level may change over time in the same individual and chronic condition. For instance, Fig. 2 illustrates how the ICF classification could be applied to hypertensive heart disease with heart failure. The figure shows the most significant categories of body functions and structure, activities and participation, and environmental factors related to heart disease, based on the empirical evidence for a core set of related CVD [8]. All the elements have their classification code, except for personal factors, which are not classified in ICF. This example also illustrates how core sets of ICF can be used for specific chronic conditions to monitor the functioning of older people in a standard way.

Specifically, ICF enables data collection on levels of functioning and disability in a consistent and comparable manner in prevention and rehabilitation medicine [9]. Furthermore, given the broad scope of ICF, core sub-sets are continually being developed and tested for specific purposes, such as the ICF Rehabilitation Sets [10], which could also be used in interventions for chronic conditions in older adults. Therefore, ICF offers a standard classification to monitor the functional evolution of older people with these and other chronic conditions, many of which are co-occurring. Indeed, various reports estimate the comorbidity prevalence in economically advanced countries for people aged 65 years and over to be around 50%, with cardiovascular diseases (CVD), Alzheimer's disease (AD) and depression being among the most common chronic conditions [11]. Moreover, CVD, AD, and depression can even lead to or be aggravated by accidental falls in older adults.

That being the case, CVD, AD, depression, and falls form an interesting example of a comorbid group of conditions because they are prevalent in older age, they disturb both physical and mental wellbeing, and there is a significant association among them.

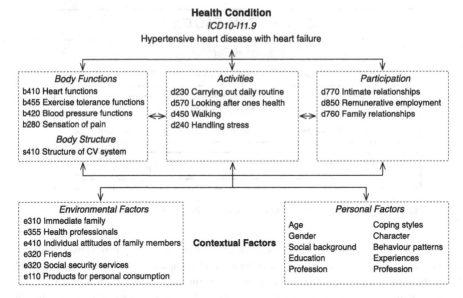

Fig. 2. Example of an ICF classification for a CVD condition

For instance, CVD and AD often lead to depression [12], with an incidence of around 25% in people with dementia [13]. Still, the association between AD and depression can be very complex, as depression is considered both a symptom of and a risk factor for AD [14]. Conversely, several studies have determined that depression is also a major risk factor for the development of CVD [15]. For instance, rates of strokes in older people can be 2.3 to 2.7 times higher in people with high levels of depression [16]. Gender may be also a significant risk factor for these conditions. For example, women are more likely to suffer depression than men, especially in older age [17]. The prevalence of AD is 40–60% among women aged 30 and over; among men the proportion increases from around 20% at age 30 to around 70% at ages 95 and over [18].

Constant intellectual, social and physical activities reduce the risk of CVD, AD and depression [19]. However, falls with injury, which are common among older adults, may hamper such activities. Thirty per cent of people over 65 and 50% of those over 80 fall annually, with women having a double lifetime risk of fracture compared to men, mainly due to osteoporosis [20]. This prevalence of falls is caused by physical, sensory, and cognitive changes associated with aging. During a longitudinal study on the main consequences and risk factors among older fallers, it was found that more than one-third suffered functional decline after falling [21]. In addition, female gender, higher medication use, depression symptoms and fall injuries were the most significant risk factors for functional decline after falling. Nonetheless, it is important that intellectual, social and physical activities continue to be carried on before, during, and after the onset of chronic conditions in older age. For this reason, interventions should induce positive behavioral changes that stimulate these activities and that promote a healthy lifestyle.

Incidentally, ICF mentions the importance of lifestyle and health-related habits (HrH) as personal determinants, but it does not offer their precise definition. To fill this gap, the Spanish Association for the Scientific Study of Healthy Aging has developed a taxonomy for the evaluation of HrH in primary care, in the context of the project eVital [22]. This taxonomy was composed by a panel of experts and is based on the conceptual model of ICF. The experts agreed on six main HrH categories for health evaluation: diet/exercise, vitality/stress, sleep, cognition, substance use, and other health habits. Of these main HrH, three are directly linked to motivation to change and should be the target of behavioral change techniques (diet/exercise, substance use, and other risk habits); the other three are less related but its monitoring is important nonetheless (cognition, vitality/stress, and sleep). In this regard, and thanks to the increase in commercial interest on Internet of Things (IoT) health monitoring technology for older people, it is now feasible to monitor and collect sufficient health-related data to predict outcomes and personalize health interventions.

3 Technologies and Strategies for Health Monitoring and Intervention

The IoT is a paradigm that considers the pervasiveness of a variety of objects connected via wire or wirelessly, which interact with each other to offer new services in creating a smart environment. In recent years, the convergence to ubiquitous services envisioned by the IoT has been accelerated by the massive adoption of smartphones, which act as hubs for many of the current connected objects. Indeed, the smartphone has become the key for IoT-based health services beyond the current concept of mobile technology for healthcare (mHealth). Given the immense market opportunities, mobile personal health monitoring (PHM) has attracted the interest of Google, Apple, and Microsoft. Each one of these companies has started offering its own ecosystem of health-related platforms, PHM services, and wearable devices and technologies. Besides, several other companies offer related (and compatible) products and services, such as consumer wearable devices, Global Positioning System (GPS) tracking, smart weight balances, and other non-wearable devices to monitor personal health and behavior.

These technologies could improve the current approaches to Remote Patient Monitoring (RPM): to collect, transmit, and evaluate the patient's health data; then to notify stakeholders when a problem based on the evaluation is detected, and eventually to intervene with an appropriate treatment or to modify a HrH. RPM is not necessarily focused on older people, but it has been integrated into the broader concept of Ambient Assisted Living (AAL), which allows older people to live in complete or partial autonomy. Moreover, AAL can aid in preventing, curing, and improving the health status of older adults [23]. The data collected from AAL systems can be integrated into the vast health system records, which could be used to automatically learn and make decisions [24]. Furthermore, predictive analytics, using innovative statistical models and techniques, allow analyzing such huge volumes of data to make predictions about the future [25].

The use of predictive and intelligent data models has many applications in healthcare, ranging from metabolic modeling, gene expression, quality of care assessment, and processing from domestic monitoring systems [26]. Current risk score and models can be automatized to predict the risk of developing certain conditions or their worsening. For instance, SCORE (Systematic COronary Risk Evaluation) is a risk scoring system used in the clinical management of cardiovascular risk in Europe to estimate fatal CVD events over a ten-year period [27]. InterHeart is a more geographically wide study, from which the InterHeart Modifiable Risk Score was developed and validated for an international population [28]. Most interestingly, new predictive models are being developed thanks to domestic monitoring systems, such as using machine learning for early detection and prediction of illness in older people [29]. In this context, machine learning refers to computers that can learn and make predictions from data without an explicit program. This is in contrast to experts systems, in which decisions are made according to an algorithm based on the knowledge of experts in the given domain, also used to asses the health status of older people [30]. Both approaches can be used in combination or under different scenarios, although machine learning is particularly apt for prediction when huge volumes of data are available.

ICT also allows us to monitor and improve the level of functioning and participation through interactive activities. Some examples of interactive activities are e-mail, web browsing and videogames. The last example is frequently related to virtual reality (VR), an immersive computer multimodal environment. There are different degrees of immersion in the Reality-Virtuality continuum, ranging from none (real environment) to fully immersive (virtual environment), with mixed reality (MR) in between. Naturally, one of the main advantages of immersive VR activities is the possibility of completely adapting the virtual environment of the user and thus offer a personalized experience to monitor or induce a change in HrH. Interest in VR has recently spiked, given that competitive commercial solutions are becoming available to individual consumers. These range from simple add-ons for smartphones (Google Cardboard and Samsung Gear VR), to much more advanced headsets for videogame consoles (PlayStation VR), personal computers (HTC Vive and Oculus Rift), or even smartphones (Google Daydream). Microsoft also works on an immersive headset, HoloLens, intended for augmented reality applications. This commercial expansion will certainly benefit the development of VR for healthcare, with many applications from medical visualization to rehabilitation therapy and serious games.

Serious games are interactive games that are specifically designed to elicit a positive change in the player, such as HrH, including physical and mental wellbeing [31]. For instance, *exer-gaming*, in which the gameplay involves significant physical exercise, can help older people with depression, balance issues, dementia, and CVD. Other kind of serious games can also improve cognitive control in older age [32]. On the other hand, in gamification, game design elements are used in a non-game context [33] to engage people in certain activities by making them entertaining and rewarding, based on intrinsic and extrinsic motivators. For example, an activity gameplay could use narrative elements to entertain, and mechanics could be based on any combination of skill, luck, and strategy. Games and gamified activities can be played alone (single-player) or with others (multi-player), either cooperatively or competitively, or both. In addition, game-based activities can complement traditional AAL systems to enhance the autonomy of older people at home [34].

4 Pervasive Predictive Analytics for Healthy Aging

Based on the benefits of the aforementioned concepts, we propose a pervasive ICT-based conceptual model to monitor, analyze, predict and improve older people's functioning levels and HrH for the prevention and rehabilitation of chronic conditions. This framework would provide data-driven personalized activities and recommendations that are accessible and adaptive to older people. The objectives of this framework are: (1) to promote self-management of prevention and rehabilitation; (2) to provide tools and mechanisms that aid in care provided by close relationships (e.g., family and friends); (3) to enable a better understanding of older people's health by the community (e.g., medical personnel, researchers, policy makers); (4) and to encourage the older individual's participation in society. This framework consists of four main parts: Remote Monitoring (RM), Predictive Analytics (PA), a User Online Platform (UOP), and a set of Interactive Activities (IA). Key risk indicators (KRI) would be selected according to the corresponding predictive models for the target conditions and factors. These KRI refer to health determinants and the functioning level of the users measured through the interactive activities (Fig. 3).

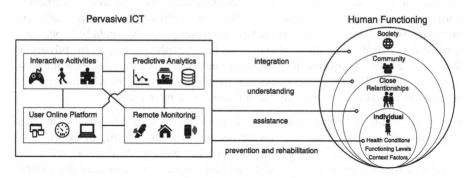

Fig. 3. Conceptual model of the proposed approach for healthy aging through pervasive ICT

Most data would be collected unobtrusively via RM, using sensors for domestic and personal use, such as fixed and wearable sensors. Other data would be collected via the interactive activities themselves, such as the performance of a given VR rehabilitation exercise. The UOP would also allow collecting other KRI, such as periodic self-assessment and risk score questionnaires, and it would allow the end users or authorized third parties (e.g., family and physicians) to monitor the current health status and receive alerts. The UOP should be user-friendly, accessible and available from both desktop and mobile devices. The UOP would also be the gateway for the set of IA and related KRI. At the beginning, the end users would have access to a common set of activities designed to maintain the overall levels of physical and mental wellbeing related to the users' age. As the health determinants, health status, and HrH of the end users evolve, the interactive activities would automatically adapt according to the analysis and prediction made by the system. To engage and entertain end users, many of these tasks would consist on activities such as MR videogames and gamified activities, besides non-game activities like online social media and other kinds of interpersonal communication. The intention is to stimulate social participation and increase the interest of the users in intellectual and physical activities to incorporate positive HrH, reducing the risk of chronic conditions. All of the end users' data from the RM, IA, and UOP would be harmonized for PA to further personalize these parts of the system.

PA would be used to analyze and detect physical or behavioral changes, based on the predictive models. With this approach, specific risks might be minimized as soon as they are detected by the system. At the same time, the progress or regress of rehabilitation therapies could be evaluated as they are applied. If the system detects significant risks or a decrease in functioning levels, an alert would be emitted to the concerned end user, close relationships, and medical personnel. Although the system would automatically monitor and personalize these aspects, it is still crucial to ease the involvement of other key stakeholders. For this reason, the UOP would provide access and ease the daily tasks of authorized care providers (physicians, nurses, etc.) and caregivers (family, friends, etc.) to follow the health evolution of the end users. Other authorized third parties could also have access to anonymized data for research, statistics and management purposes. For example, researchers could analyze the data to study and discover patterns, causes and effects of health conditions across different categories, or discover possible socio-behavioral patterns, etc. As might be expected, a strict access control policy for each role would be established to respect the privacy of the patients and other sensitive information, in compliance with the corresponding local legislation. Regarding the stakeholders that would directly interact with the different parts of the framework, we identify the following four main roles:

- End user: This is the main stakeholder in the framework. The end user is an older person who wants to improve his or her health status by improving the own health-related habits, either for prevention or rehabilitation. The end user is also the primary stakeholder in the RM part of the framework, which automatically collects the necessary health-related data. In addition, the end user can interact with the UOP, either to collect additional data or for self-monitoring, as well as a gateway to the IA.

- Caregivers: A caregiver is a person who helps the end user in his or her activities in daily life. Usually the caregiver is a close relationship, such as a family member, but sometimes it can also be a paid person. Caregivers would be able to accompany the end user in their utilization of the RM and execution of IA, and they would also have personalized access to the UOP to monitor or receive alerts on their corresponding end user.

- Care providers: These are health professionals that offer preventive, curative, or rehabilitative health services to the end user. As with the caregivers, care providers would have a personalized access and alerts regarding the data of their end user or group of end users through the UOP. However, care providers would have access to a more comprehensive set of functionalities to monitor the health of their end users.

• Researchers: The researchers are professionals from different scientific disciplines (e.g., clinicians, gerontologist, psychologist, sociologists, and computer scientists) who are interested in the inner workings and improvement of all of the parts of the framework, particularly the tuning of the PA.

Of course, in addition to these roles, there are other important stakeholders (e.g., policy makers) that determine the health status of older people, but these are influenced by the four roles identified above, instead of interacting directly with the parts of the framework. Besides, the proposed framework is also independent of the underlying approaches, technologies, and implementation chosen. The RM could be implemented using Bluetooth, ZigBee or other standard for wireless sensor networks; the UOP could be accessed via native applications for mobile systems, desktop environments, or special units; the IA could be serious games or other gamified activities across the reality-virtuality continuum; and the PA could use diverse approaches (or combinations of) for predictive modeling and analysis such as expert systems and machine learning. These technologies and standards are rapidly evolving; nonetheless, we believe that the principles of the proposed framework serve as a high-level conceptual model for future research.

5   Conclusions

We have described how chronic conditions in older age are prevalent and interlinked, the benefits of using international standards to classify the functioning level of these conditions, and how ICT could be applied to prevent and rehabilitate through pervasive predictive analytics. Our proposed data-driven approach is a cohesive combination of these concepts that aims to move forward current implementations of PHR and AAL in older people. Nonetheless, several issues need to be tackled before a successful implementation based on this approach. For instance, there are no universally adapted open standards for health data, IoT and VR technology, although academia, industry, and standardization bodies are working on this issue. In addition, the disparity around the world concerning legal frameworks regarding data protection and privacy is another critical issue, but one that is beyond the scope of the present work. Given that our approach implicates the collection of highly sensitive data and the profiling of older people's functioning, we need to implement secure transmission and to control access to these data to avoid their misuse. Despite these current shortcomings, we believe that our framework could be used as a conceptual basis for future research on prevention and rehabilitation of chronic conditions in older age through pervasive, predictive, and personalized health solutions.

References

1. Karlamangla, A., Tinetti, M., Guralnik, J., Studenski, S., Wetle, T., Reuben, D.: Comorbidity in older adults: nosology of impairment, diseases, and conditions. J. Gerontol. Ser. A Biol. Sci. Med. Sci. **62**(3), 296–300 (2007)
2. Kirkpatrick, K.: Sensors for seniors. Commun. ACM **57**(12), 17–19 (2014)
3. Coyle, H., Traynor, V., Solowij, N.: Computerized and virtual reality cognitive training for individuals at high risk of cognitive decline: systematic review of the literature. Am. J. Geriatr. Psychiatry **23**(4), 335–359 (2015)
4. Buzzi, M.C., Buzzi, M., Trujillo, A. (eds.): Healthy aging through pervasive predictive analytics for prevention and rehabilitation of chronic conditions. In: Proceedings of the 3rd 2015 Workshop on ICTs for improving Patients Rehabilitation Research Techniques. ACM (2015)
5. Baccarelli, A., Rienstra, M., Benjamin, E.J.: Cardiovascular epigenetics basic concepts and results from animal and human studies. Circ. Cardiovasc. Genet. **3**(6), 567–573 (2010)
6. Peel, N.M., McClure, R.J., Bartlett, H.P.: Behavioral determinants of healthy aging. Am. J. Prev. Med. **28**(3), 298–304 (2005)
7. Rowe, J.W., Kahn, R.L.: Successful aging. Gerontologist **37**(4), 433–440 (1997)
8. Cieza, A., Stucki, A., Geyh, S., Berteanu, M., Quittan, M., Simon, A., et al.: ICF core sets for chronic ischaemic heart disease. J. Rehabil. Med. **36**, 94–99 (2004)
9. Stucki, G., Ewert, T., Cieza, A.: Value and application of the ICF in rehabilitation medicine. Disabil. Rehabil. **24**(17), 932–938 (2002)
10. Prodinger, B., Cieza, A., Oberhauser, C., Bickenbach, J., Üstün, T.B., Chatterji, S., et al.: Toward the international classification of functioning, disability and health (ICF) rehabilitation set: a minimal generic set of domains for rehabilitation as a health strategy. Arch. Phys. Med. Rehabil. **97**, 875–884 (2016)
11. Nolte, E., McKee, M.: Caring for people with chronic conditions: a health system perspective. In: A Health System Perspective. McGraw-Hill International, Berkshire (2008)
12. Blazer, D.G.: Depression in late life: review and commentary. J. Gerontol. Med. Sci. **58A**, 249–265 (2003)
13. Lobo, A., Saz, P., Marcos, G., Día, J., De-la-Cámara, C.: The prevalence of dementia and depression in the elderly community in a southern European population: The Zaragoza study. Arch. Gen. Psychiatry **52**(6), 497–506 (1995)
14. Devanand, D.P., Sano, M., Tang, M., et al.: Depressed mood and the incidence of alzheimer's disease in the elderly living in the community. Arch. Gen. Psychiatry **53**(2), 175–182 (1996)
15. Musselman, D.L., Evans, D.L., Nemeroff, C.B.: The relationship of depression to cardiovascular disease: epidemiology, biology, and treatment. Arch. Gen. Psychiatry **55**(7), 580–592 (1998)
16. Simonsick, E.M., Wallace, R.B., Blazer, D.G., Berkman, L.F.: Depressive symptomatology and hypertension-associated morbidity and mortality in older adults. Psychosom. Med. **57**(5), 427–435 (1995)
17. Mukkala, M., O'Sullivan, C., Lowes, S.: Mental Health Indicators and Data in EU Member States. Scottish Development Centre for Mental Health, Edinburg (2008)
18. Knapp, M., Prince, M., Albanese, E., Banerjee, S., Dhanasiri, S., Fernandez, J., et al.: Dementia UK, p. 7. Alzheimer's Society, London (2007)
19. Prevention CfDCa: The State of Aging and Health in America 2013, Atlanta (2013)

20. World Health Organization: What are the main risk factors for falls amongst older people and what are the most effective interventions to prevent these falls? Regional Office for Europe, Copenhagen (2004)

21. Stel, V.S., Smit, J.H., Pluijm, S.M., Lips, P.: Consequences of falling in older men and women and risk factors for health service use and functional decline. Age Ageing 33(1), 58–65 (2004)

22. Salvador-Carulla, L., Alonso, F., Gomez, R., Walsh, C.O., Almenara, J., Ruiz, M., et al.: Basic concepts in the taxonomy of health-related behaviors, habits and lifestyle. Int. J. Environ. Res. Pub. Health 10(5), 1963–1976 (2013)

23. Rashidi, P., Mihailidis, A.: A survey on ambient-assisted living tools for older adults. IEEE J. Biomed. Health Inform. 17(3), 579–590 (2013)

24. Ainsworth, J., Buchan, I.: Combining health data uses to ignite health system learning. Methods Inf. Med. 54(6), 479–487 (2015)

25. McAfee, A., Brynjolfsson, E.: Big data: the management revolution. Harv. Bus. Rev. 90:60–68, 128 (2012)

26. Peek, N., Swift, S.: Intelligent data analysis for knowledge discovery, patient monitoring and quality assessment. Methods Inf. Med. 51(4), 318 (2012)

27. Conroy, R., Pyörälä, K., Ae, F., Sans, S., Menotti, A., De Backer, G., et al.: Estimation of ten-year risk of fatal cardiovascular disease in Europe: the SCORE project. Eur. Heart J. 24 (11), 987–1003 (2003)

28. McGorrian, C., Yusuf, S., Islam, S., Jung, H., Rangarajan, S., Avezum, A. et al.: Estimating modifiable coronary heart disease risk in multiple regions of the world: the INTERHEART modifiable risk score. Eur. Heart J. (2010). doi:10.1093/eurheartj/ehq448

29. Popescu, M., Mahnot, A.: Early illness recognition using in-home monitoring sensors and multiple instance learning. Methods Inf. Med. 51(4), 359 (2012)

30. Iliffe, S., Kharicha, K., Harari, D., Swift, C., Stuck, A.: Health risk appraisal for older people in general practice using an expert system: a pilot study. Health Soc. Care Community 13(1), 21–29 (2005)

31. McCallum, S.: Gamification and serious games for personalized health. Stud. Health Technol. Inform. 177, 85–96 (2012)

32. Basak, C., Boot, W.R., Voss, M.W., Kramer, A.F.: Can training in a real-time strategy video game attenuate cognitive decline in older adults? Psychol. Aging 23(4), 765 (2008)

33. Deterding, S., Dixon, D., Khaled, R., Nacke, L. (eds.): From game design elements to gamefulness: defining gamification. In: Proceedings of the 15th International Academic MindTrek Conference: Envisioning Future Media Environments. ACM (2011)

34. Leonhardt, S., Kassel, S., Randow, A., Teich, T.: Learning in the context of an ambient assisted living apartment: Including methods of serious gaming. In: Motta, G., Wu, B. (eds.) Software Engineering Education for a Global E-Service Economy. Progress in IS, pp. 49–55. Springer, Cham (2014)

A Virtual System for Balance Control Assessment at Home

Matteo Spezialetti[1](✉), Daniela Iacoviello[2], Andrea Petracca[1],
and Giuseppe Placidi[1]

[1] A²VI_Lab, c/o Department of Life, Health and Environmental Sciences,
University of L'Aquila, Via Vetoio, 67100 L'aquila, Italy
{matteo.spezialetti,andrea.petracca}@graduate.univaq.it,
giuseppe.placidi@univaq.it
[2] Department of Computer, Control and Management Engineering Antonio Ruberti,
Sapienza University of Rome, Via Ariosto 25, 00185 Rome, Italy
iacoviello@dis.uniroma1.it

Abstract. Postural stability is often compromised in many pathological
states and decreases with age. In clinical practice, an objective tool for
balance control at home is fundamental. Recently, virtual tools, based on
the use of depth cameras, have been presented. In this paper, a virtual
system for balance control assessment is presented and used to implement
a virtual task for balance tracking in real time at home. The usability
of the tool is assessed through some experimental data collected by 6
healthy elderly people, that used the system and evaluated it through a
questionnaire. Results are reported and discussed.

Keywords: Postural balance · Rehabilitation · Virtual reality

1 Introduction

Balance control is the ability to maintaining the body Center Of Mass (COM)
within its limits of stability. This capability, fundamental for controlling body
movement, decreases with age [1] and could be compromised by many pathologies
[2–4]. Both for diagnostic purposes (a timely control of the postural stability
reduction could prevent the risk of falls) and for assessing therapeutic progresses
an objective and quantitative postural balance assessment at home is needed.
Recently, the effectiveness of a new generation of virtual instruments, exercises
and practices for rehabilitation have been studied and developed [5–14].

The evolution of the postural sway can be defined statically, if measurements
are made while the subject tries to remain still standing, or dynamically, if the
measurements are made under the effects of tasks aiming at changing balance
conditions (important to assess the maintenance of an unstable equilibrium) [15].
Obviously, systems allowing dynamic measurements are also usable for static
studies.

Postural sway could be estimated starting from kinetic or kinematics parameters. The kinetic information include the excursion of the Center of Pressure

© Springer International Publishing AG 2017
H.M. Fardoun et al. (Eds.): REHAB 2015, CCIS 665, pp. 12–25, 2017.
https://doi.org/10.1007/978-3-319-69694-2_2

(COP), applied to a support surface, and measured by means of clinical force platforms [16] or low-cost commercial instruments, like for example the Wii Balance [17].

The kinematic data could be used to estimate the spatial position of the Center of Mass and, consequently, its vertical projection on the ground, the Center of Gravity (COG). It could be measured by using wearable inertial sensors [18] or optical motion analysis [19]. In particular, in [19] a low-cost tool for COM/COG assessment, based on a TOF camera has been described.

During a virtual balance task, the COG excursions have been recorded and compared with the movements done by COP, acquired by means of a force platform. Results have shown that this tool was able to assess the sway of the human body also in dynamic conditions. The system had a lower dynamic range than a physical force platform, mainly due to the difference between COG and COP [20]. However, those differences were more evident in the Medio-Lateral (ML) direction of the subject movements than in the Antero-Posterior (AP) direction [19].

This systematic error was produced because the Field Of View (FOV) of the camera was partial. Moreover, to ensure a real-time response, the model of the human body was approximated by a reduced set of spheres over the depth map. In [21,22], a refinement of the system has been proposed to overcome these limitations by using a mirror. In fact, the mirror allowed the focusing of occluded portions of the body and could be used both with a Structured Light (SL) Camera (e.g. Kinect 1) or with a TOF Camera (e.g. Kinect 2). The use of the mirror, instead of an additional depth sensing camera, had two advantages: it was cheap and it avoided multiple-camera synchronization and high-frequency acquisition. The present paper describes a balance tracking software to assess the balance control ability in elderly people at home; the application is integrated with the system [21,22] and tested on a set of 6 healthy elderly people.

The paper is organized as follows: Sect. 2 describes the proposed system, briefly reports the depth map generation process for TOF or SL cameras, summarizes the balance assessment system, and describes the application for the dynamic and real time balance tracking. Section 3 shows and discusses some experimental results regarding the system usability, whereas in Sect. 4 some conclusions are presented.

2   System Design

The proposed system was designed to fit the requirements of three stakeholders: the beneficiary, the therapists, and the caregivers. Potential beneficiaries are, mainly, aged people but also people with balance deficits derived from neurological or musculoskeletal disorder (in the following we use also the term "user" to identify the "beneficiary", though a user of the system could also be a therapist or a caregiver). Regarding the beneficiaries, the system has to be easy to use, presuming that most of them probably are unskilled of computers. In fact, the system must be usable at home without external help. Moreover, the system should elaborate the current balance session and exhibit to the user the outcome of the session itself (in case of positive result, the system should show a positive message to the user whereas in case of negative result, the system should signal a warning). Finally, the system has to be safe, in the sense that it has to be easily set by qualified therapists, according to the users capacities and needs, but it must not be allowed to the users to modify the system setting, in order to avoid dangerous situations (the system could become the cause of falls!). According to the therapist stakeholder, besides the possibility of setting, the system has to store raw data of executed sessions, and to furnish simply usable tools for rapid data retrieving, analysis, and visualization. Referred to the caregivers, the main target is to be informed regarding the regular usage of the system (jumping a planned session could imply a warning situation) and of the results of the monitoring activity (a negative outcome of the current session would imply a warning message).

The system architecture is structured in order to be deployed on up to three different machines. As shown in Fig. 1, four main components can be identified: (a) the depth camera and the mirror, essential for the COG assessment; (b) the installation machine used to calibrate the system, equipped with the software necessary to collect both the RGB and the depth map from the camera and the Matlab environment with the Camera Calibration Toolbox [23]; (c) the server machine, equipped with the driver and the libraries for the communication with the depth map, that hosted both the COG computation module and the web application for the static and the dynamic posturography; (d) the client machine, where only a web browser has to be installed.

2.1   Integration of a Depth Camera with a Mirror

The depth sensing camera can be plugged, by means of an USB connection, both to the server or to the installation machine, depending on the state in which the system is (calibration state or balance tool execution state). As demonstrated in [19], the camera is used in conjunction with a mirror in order to improve the COG assessment accuracy, by retrieving information about the hidden surface of the user body.

TOF sensors are composed by an emitter and a sensor matrix that work at near infrared (NIR) light frequencies. As shown in Fig. 2a, by enlightening the scene with a light (by means of the emitter E), modulated in amplitude by a *sine* of frequency f_{mod}, and measuring the phase shift (φ_{shift}) between the emitted and the reflected signal (captured by the sensor S), it is possible to compute the distance of an object O from the matrix plane and the depth map of the scene [24]. Then, being note the horizontal and the vertical fields of view of the camera, it is possible to compute the spatial coordinates of a point $O = (x_O, y_O, z_O)$, referred to a three-dimensional Cartesian coordinates system, typically centered on the middle of the camera sensor.

Figure 2b, shows that the placement of a mirror in the scene allows the indirect observation of an object, through its reflection: the light, reflected by the mirror, hits the object O and it is detected by the sensor S as if there is a

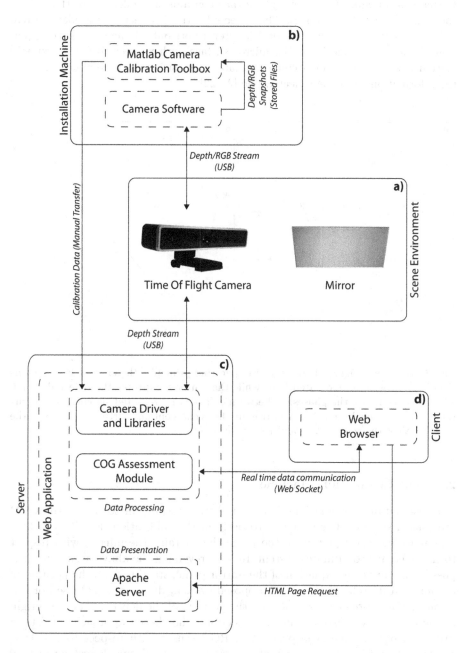

Fig. 1. Architecture diagram of the system, composed by four main components: (a) the TOF camera and the mirror, (b) the installation machine (c) the server machine, (d) the client machine.

virtual space behind the mirror plane that contains the reflection of the object, the sensor and the emitter E. The reflected virtual object VO is like the real object O, seen by a virtual sensor VS, after a horizontal image flip. If the equation of the plane containing the mirror surface with respect to the coordinate system is known, it is possible to estimate the position of the real object using the information from the reflected one [21, 22].

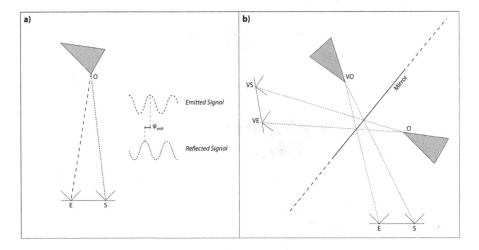

Fig. 2. a) Time of flight (TOF) camera operating principle: the emitter E enlightens the object O with a modulated light while the sensor S captures the reflected signal, allowing to compute the phaseshift between emitted and reflected signals. (b) the virtual space created by placing a mirror in the scene contains virtual versions of the emitter (VE), the sensor (VS) and the object (VO).

2.2   The Installation Machine

The installation machine function is to allow a technician to set up the COG acquisition system. It is designed to perform the calibration described in [22], that is to find the equation of the plane the contains the mirror, with respect to the reference coordinates system. Indeed, reversing the above argument, it is possible to derive the equation of the mirror plane, starting from the position of a point and its reflection. In the proposed system, due to the TOF sensor low resolution, it is preferred to calculate the position of the depth sensor (the origin of the coordinates system) and its reflection. The chosen approach consists in two main phases: first, the position of RGB sensor with respect to the TOF sensor is found, by using a set of images of a special chessboard formed by alternating opaque and reflective squares visible from both sensors; second, a set of images of a chessboard, seen both directly and through its reflection, is used to calculate the reciprocal positions of the two RGB sensors (the real and the virtual one seen through the mirror). As shown in Fig. 3, the same image is used to represent the views of the object from both the cameras, after a horizontal flip. These information allows to compute the reciprocal position of the two TOF sensors and the plane equation. In this phase, the coordinates of a pixel in the depth map, belonging to the ground, are calculated in order to store the height H of the camera from the floor. In the proposed version of the system, the calibration process is performed by using the Camera Calibration Toolbox [23], and produces a binary output file containing the plane coefficients value and the camera distance from the floor H, manually transferred to the server machine. In future developments, this step will be implemented in proprietary software tool, that will simplify operations needed during the process, by means of a wizard, allowing the therapist or the caregiver to set up the system. For this reason the technician is not identified as stakeholder.

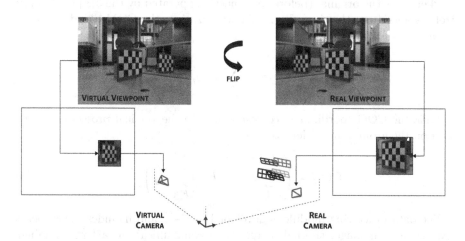

Fig. 3. The couple of images used for the calibration between the real and the virtual RGB cameras: one is obtained as the horizontal flip of the other. The result of the calibration test, indicating the mutual position of real camera with respect to the virtual one, is also shown (below).

2.3   The Server Machine

The server machine hosts the web application that executes two main modules, data processing tool and data presentation tool. The first manages the communication with the TOF camera and is equipped with the implementation of the COG assessment algorithm described in [22]. Two phases are required, for each frame, in order to obtain the COG: the 3D positioning and the COG evaluation.

The 3D positioning aims at computing, for each frame, the spatial coordinates of the body surface by using the pixels allowing both to the direct foreground and to the reflected one. First, each point of the foreground is determined in the 3D coordinates system (direct and reflected images are managed in the same way). Second, it is marked as "real", if belonging to the same half-space of the system origin, "virtual" elsewhere (this operation is simplified by reserving a region of scene to the mirror). Finally, the reflection with respect to the mirror plane is applied to each virtual pixel.

For the COG evaluation a weight-based approach is used in order to normalize the pixel contribution to the COG evaluation, proportionally to the body surface covered by it (a closer pixel would have a lower contribution with respect to a farther one). Since the surface covered by a pixel increases like the square of the distance, for each pixel i belonging to the foreground F, the considered weight is:

$$w_i = \frac{d_i^2}{\sum_{j \in F} d_j^2}.$$ (1)

where d_i is the original (before the reflection operated by the 3D positioning) pixel distance from the camera. After normalization, the COM coordinates are computed as follows:

$$COM = \left(\sum_{j \in F} w_j x_j, \sum_{j \in F} w_j y_j, \sum_{j \in F} w_j z_j \right).$$ (2)

while the COG coordinates, corresponding to the vertical projection of the COM on the ground, are calculated as:

$$COG = \left(\sum_{j \in F} w_j x_j, -H, \sum_{j \in F} w_j z_j \right).$$ (3)

The data processing module is developed in C++ and includes a websocket server able to manage, through a real time communication, a large numbers of messages exchanged from and to the client. It must synchronize the information processed by the COG algorithm and consumed (and presented) by the client itself. WebSockets protocol [25] has been selected for the proposed system because it provides a consistent latency reduction and avoids unnecessary network traffic, if compared to polling and long-polling solutions that are used to simulate a full-duplex connection by maintaining two connections. Thus the WebSockets represent a standard for bi-directional real time communication/applications [26].

Data presentation module exploits the features of the installed Apache Server [27] and is used to deploy the graphic interface pages and to handle the http requests from the web-browser.

The above design, following the classic client-server architecture, allows to deploy the modules for data processing on the server machine, thus limiting the role of the client to simply host a web browser. This choice has been successfully used also in the interface design of a communication tool for impaired people [28].

Figure 4 shows the two possible execution scenarios of the system: the first (Fig. 4(a)) is designed for static posturography, the second (Fig. 4(b)) is used to execute a combined static/dynamic posturography chain.

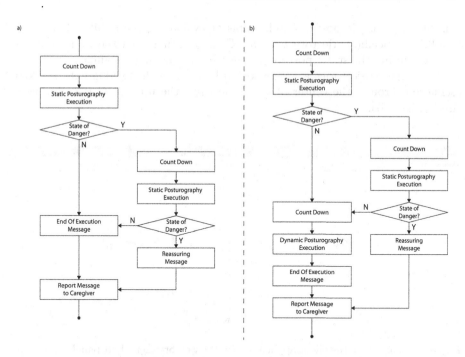

Fig. 4. Block Diagram of the two possible COG control scenarios: (a) while maintaining a static position; (b) by using a multiple task consisting both in maintaining a static position and tracking a moving target (for safety issues, the tracking task is allowed only if the static position maintenance has a positive outcome).

In both scenarios the tool is used as a control instrument, in order to periodically check the balance control of the subject and notify the caregiver of daily executions and progresses and, above all, of potential dangerous balance states recorded by the system. The balance check is performed through the execution of up to two static posturography sessions. If both of them result in a warning, by exceeding the displacement limit either for AP or ML swaying, the system displays a reassuring message that is intended to calm down the subject and to make him sit down, without worry him: "Please wait until computation is complete. Take a seat and rest for a minute". At the end of the scenarios, a system call is executed, in order to report to the caregiver about the state of the subject. The effects of the call can be defined by modifying the type and the content of the file indexed in the setting (it could be, for example, a batch file or an executable). Thus, several strategies could be used to report, like sending an email, doing a http request or exploiting an SMS provider.

Static posturography is designed to assess the ability of the user to maintain fixed his COG. The user has to keep is arms along the body and his feet joined, staying as still as possible.

In this case the user interface contains just the representation of the user COG position (drawn as a circle) and its movement on the horizontal plane

(Fig. 5(a)). Dynamic posturography aims at evaluating the ability of the user to follow a specific trajectory with his COG, starting from the same position assumed during the static posturography and just moving his ankles.

The target trajectories are represented by a gun sight moving with random oscillations around the center of the scene while the user COG is drawn as a circle (Fig. 5(b)).

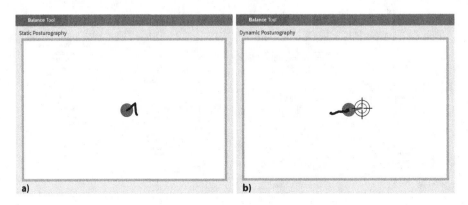

Fig. 5. Screenshots of the client application (in the web browser). Left panel (a) reports the static posturography window, containing the representation of the user COG position (red circle) and its trajectory on the horizontal plane (black stroke). Right panel (b) represents the dynamic posturography window: the target is represented by a gun sight moving, with a pre-determined trajectory (the last two seconds of the followed path is indicated by a green stroke), around the center of the scene and the user COG is drawn as a red circle with the last 2 s of its trajectory (black stroke). (Color figure online)

The whole system is designed to require the minimum possible amount of operations that the user has to perform to use the system and, at the same time, to avoid the possibility of wrong setting that an unskilled user could produce. A text file stored on the server machine defines the values of parameters used in the application: the scenario that has to be executed (COG control both maintaining a static position or tracking a moving target), the task duration (both for static and dynamic tasks), the delay between the execution of the application and the beginning of the task, the AP or the ML values of displacement that, if exceeded during the static posturography, has to be considered dangerous and, finally, the path of the file that has to be executed in case of a balance warning situation.

Data recorded during the executions are stored in the server machine in order to give to the therapist the possibility of analyzing and comparing them in future.

3   System Evaluation

The proposed system has been evaluated, in terms of user usability, by performing a set of test sessions.

The experimental settings was composed of a TOF camera [29], located at 3.5 m from the expected subject location and 1.45 m from the floor, and a squared mirror (1.5 m sided), positioned with its center at 4.5 m from the camera and 2.35 m from the floor. The mirror was inclined by 50° with respect to the vertical position. The machines acting as server, client and installation coincided to the same computer, an Intel i7 (2.3 GHz) with 4 GB of RAM and Windows 7 (64bit). The web browser that played the client role has been executed in full-screen option and projected from the ceil on the floor, just in front of the user position, in order to increase the feeling of augmented reality for the user. The executed scenario was composed by 90 s long static and dynamic tasks (Fig. 4(b) and settings included a delay before each posturography test of 15 s and a 5 cm displacement warning value, both for AP and ML directions.

Experimental data has been collected by 6 healthy voluntary subjects, 3 women and 3 men, average age of 60.7 years (±3.2 years). The subjects had scarce or absent ability of using computers. Each participant has been summoned, the day before the test, for a brief, individual meeting, regarding the correct use of the system.

Experimental test required a list of operation that had to be performed by the subjects: (a) running the server application; (b) opening the browser and connecting to the application URL (this operation is facilitated by a shortcut icon on the desktop); (c) executing the combined sequence of task; (d) closing the browser and the server.

All the subjects have achieved to perform the dynamic task passing through the static check only once. After the session each participant has been requested to fill the SUS questionnaire [30], in order to evaluate the usability of the system. The SUS questionnaire is composed by 10 item that have to be scored in the range from 1 to 5 (meaning from "strongly disagreement" to "strongly agreement"): five items are related with a positive usability meaning (e.g. "I felt very confident using the system"), while the remaining are negative statements (e.g. "I found the system unnecessarily complex"). The final score S, ranging from 0 to 100, is computed as follows:

$$S = \left(\sum_{j \in P} (V_j - 1) + \sum_{j \in N} (5 - V_j) \right) * 2.5. \tag{4}$$

Where P and N are the set of positive and negative items respectively, and V_i is the value assigned to the statement i.

The system has been scored with 71.7 as average usability value, corresponding with quite positive overall opinion. Figure 6 summarizes the individual questionnaire results: 5 subjects have valuated the system usability with a score of 65 or above while one (Subject #5) has found the system very difficult to be used.

Since the subject had almost never experienced the use of a personal computer, most of the difficulties could be attributed to the interaction with the operating system more than with the proposed system. Indeed, both during the training session and the test session, the subject has been observed to have problem with basic operations like double-clicking on an icon or closing a window. The other subjects have considered easy or friendly the interaction with the proposed system and, though the questionnaire was strictly related to usability, some of them have pointed out that they have found funny the dynamic version of the system.

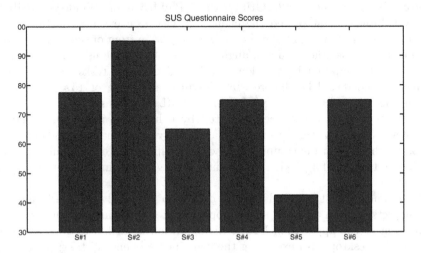

Fig. 6. Chart of the SUS questionnaire scores over the subjects. Scores axis is shown cut (from 30 to 100) for visualization purposes.

Figure 7 reports, as an example, the COG movements recorded during the Subject #1 dynamic session. The figure also shows the trajectory of the moving target (in particular, in the first and the second graphs the user trajectories are shown with continuous lines, while the target movements are represented by dotted lines). As it is possible to see from the plots, the user COG follows trajectories that includes higher frequencies components with respect to those drawn by the target (due to trembling movements). The COG trajectory also presents an obvious temporal delay (the user had to adapt his actions to the target) and greater oscillations amplitudes, because the user response to the target changes of direction was not immediate, leading him to overtake it.

Data reported are an example of the information that could be analyzed and elaborated by the therapist, by taking into account the COG movements and, in case of dynamic tasks, the position of the target.

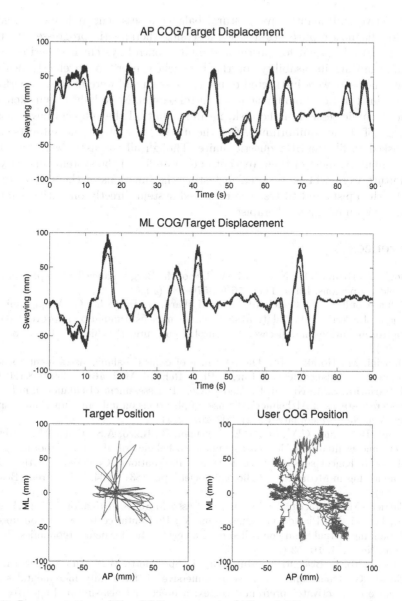

Fig. 7. Representation of the COG movements (AP and ML components) recorded and visualized by the system during a dynamic session the Subject #1. In particular, the continuous lines represent the target trajectories and the dotted lines represent the COG trajectories of the analyzed subject. In the last row the figure show the trajectories represented on the plane.

4 Conclusion

An objective and quantitative postural balance assessment at home is needed both for diagnostic purposes and for assessing therapeutic progresses. In this paper a virtual system for postural stability control system is described and tested, regarding its usability for the beneficiary users, on 6 elderly healthy people. The users were instructed to use the system and were invited to perform the combined static/dynamic balance control session. Nobody has been excluded by the dynamic session of the task, meaning that all the subjects have passed the stage of static equilibrium. After the use of the system, the subjects have been asked to fill the SUS questionnaire. Though all the users were unskilled with computers, most of them (except one) have found the system very easy to use. Future work will be devoted in testing the functions of the system to be used by therapists and to test the proposed system directly on patients under the supervision of expert therapists.

References

1. Bogle Thorbahn, L.D., Newton, R.A.: Use of the Berg Balance Test to predict falls in elderly persons. Phys. Ther. **76**(6), 576–583 (1996)
2. Colnat-Coulbois, S., Gauchard, G.C., Maillard, L., Barroche, G., Vespignani, H., Auque, J., Perrin, P.P.: Bilateral subthalamic nucleus stimulation improves balance control in Parkinson's disease. J. Neurol. Neurosurg. Psychiatry. **76**(6), 780–787 (2005)
3. Mancini, M., Horak, F.B.: The relevance of clinical balance assessment tools to differentiate balance deficits. Eur. J. Phys. Rehabil. Med. **46**(2), 239–248 (2010)
4. Kato-Narita, E.M., Nitrini, R., Radanovic, M.: Assessment of balance in mild and moderate stages of Alzheimer's disease: implications on falls and functional capacity. Arq. Neuro-Psiquiatr. **69**(2), 202–207 (2011)
5. Lange, B., Chang, C.Y., Suma, E., Newman, B., Rizzo, A.S., Bolas, M.: Development and evaluation of low cost game-based balance rehabilitation tool using the Microsoft Kinect sensor. In: 2011 Annual International Conference of the IEEE Engineering in Medicine and Biology Society, pp. 1831–1834. IEEE Press, Boston (2011)
6. Carrieri, M., Petracca, A., Lancia, S., Basso Moro, S., Brigadoi, S., Spezialetti, M., Ferrari, M., Placidi, G., Quaresima, V.: Prefrontal cortex activation upon a demanding virtual hand-controlled task: a new frontier for neuroergonomics. Front. Hum. Neurosci. **10**, 53 (2016)
7. Basso Moro, S., Bisconti, S., Muthalib, M., Spezialetti, M., Cutini, S., Ferrari, M., Placidi, G., Quaresima, V.: A semi-immersive virtual reality incremental swing balance task activates prefrontal cortex: a functional near-infrared spectroscopy study. NeuroImage **85**(1), 451–460 (2014)
8. Avola, D., Spezialetti, M., Placidi, G.: Design of an efficient framework for fast prototyping of customized human-computer interfaces and virtual environments for rehabilitation. Comput. Methods Programs Biomed. **110**(3), 490–502 (2013)
9. Petracca, A., Carrieri, M., Avola, D., Basso Moro, S., Brigadoi, S., Lancia, S., Spezialetti, M., Ferrari, M., Quaresima, V., Placidi, G.: A virtual ball task driven by forearm movements for neuro-rehabilitation. 2015 International Conference on Virtual Rehabilitation (ICVR), pp. 162–163. IEEE Press, Valencia (2015)

10. Lloréns, R., Noé, E., Naranjo, V., Borrego, A., Latorre, J., Alcañiz, M.: Tracking systems for virtual rehabilitation: objective performance vs subjective experience. A practical scenario. Sensors 15, 6586–6606 (2015)
11. Placidi, G.: A smart virtual glove for the hand telerehabilitation. Comput. Biol. Med. 37(8), 1100–1107 (2007)
12. Franchi, D., Maurizi, A., Placidi, G.: Characterization of a simmechanics model for a virtual glove rehabilitation system. In: Barneva, R.P., Brimkov, V.E., Hauptman, H.A., Natal Jorge, R.M., Tavares, J.M.R.S. (eds.) CompIMAGE 2010. LNCS, vol. 6026, pp. 141–150. Springer, Heidelberg (2010). doi:10.1007/978-3-642-12712-0_13
13. Placidi, G., Avola, D., Iacoviello, D., Cinque, L.: Overall design and implementation of the virtual glove. Comput. Biol. Med. 43(11), 1927–1940 (2013)
14. Basso Moro, S., Carrieri, M., Avola, D., Brigadoi, S., Lancia, S., Petracca, A., Spezialetti, M., Ferrari, M., Placidi, G., Quaresima, V.: A novel semi-immersive virtual reality visuo-motor task activates ventrolateral prefrontal cortex: a functional near-infrared spectroscopy study. J. Neural Eng. 13, 3 (2016)
15. Visser, J., Carpenter, M., van der Kooij, H., Bloem, B.: The clinical utility of posturography. Clin. Neurophysiol. 119(11), 2424–2436 (2008)
16. Prosperini, L., Pozzilli, C.: The clinical relevance of force platform measures in multiple sclerosis: a review. Multiple Sclerosis International, pp. 1–9 (2013)
17. Wii Balance Board. http://wiifit.com/what-is-wii-fit-plus/#balance-board
18. Bonato, P.: J. NeuroEng. Rehabil. 2, 2 (2005)
19. Placidi, G., Avola, D., Ferrari, M., Iacoviello, D., Petracca, A., Quaresima, V., Spezialetti, M.: A low-cost real time virtual system for postural stability assessment at home. Comput. Methods Programs Biomed. 117(2), 322–333 (2014)
20. Zatsiorsky, V., King, D.: An algorithm for determining gravity line location from posturographic recordings. J. Biomech. 31(2), 161–164 (1997)
21. Placidi, G., Petracca, A., Pagnani, N., Spezialetti, M., Iacoviello, D.: A virtual system for postural stability assessment based on a TOF camera and a mirror. In: Proceedings of the 3rd 2015 Workshop on ICTs for Improving Patients Rehabilitation Research Techniques, pp. 77–80. ACM, New York (2015)
22. Spezialetti, M., Iacoviello, D., Pagnani, N., Petracca, A., Placidi, G.: Mirrors and depth camera to emulate a multiple sensors environment for postural stability assessment. In: Methods of Information in Medicine (2016, submitted)
23. Camera Calibration Toolbox for Matlab. http://www.vision.caltech.edu/bouguetj/calib_doc/
24. Hansard, M., Lee, S., Choi, O., Horaud, R.P.: Time-of-Flight Cameras: Principles, Methods and Applications. Springer, London (2012). doi:10.1007/978-1-4471-4658-2
25. RFC 6455 - The WebSocket protocol. https://tools.ietf.org/html/rfc6455
26. Pimentel, V., Nickerson, B.: Communicating and displaying real-time data with websocket. IEEE Internet Comput. 16, 45–53 (2012)
27. The Apache HTTP Server Project. https://httpd.apache.org/
28. Placidi, G., Petracca, A., Spezialetti, M., Iacoviello, D.: A modular framework for EEG web based binary brain computer interfaces to recover communication abilities in impaired people. J. Med. Syst. 40, 34 (2015)
29. W20130527 SK DS311 Datasheet Recto V3.0 vectorized - SoftKinetics; c2007–2015. http://www.softkinetic.com/
30. Brooke, J.: SUS-A quick and dirty usability scale. Usability Eval. Ind. 189(194), 4–7 (1996)

Assessment of Attentional and Mnesic Processes Through Gaze Tracking Analysis: Inferences from Comparative Search Tasks Embedded in VR Serious Games

Pedro J. Rosa[1,2,3,4(✉)], Diogo Morais[1,2], Jorge Oliveira[1,2],
Pedro Gamito[1,2], Olivia Smyth[5], and Matthew Pavlovic[5]

[1] ECPV, Universidade Lusófona de Humanidades e Tecnologias,
Lisbon, Portugal
{pedro.rosa, diogo.morais,
jorge.oliveira, pedro.gamito}@ulusofona.pt
[2] School of Psychology and Life Sciences,
COPELABS–ULHT, Lisbon, Portugal
[3] Instituto Universitário de Lisboa (ISCTE-IUL), Cis-IUL, Lisbon, Portugal
[4] Centro de Investigação em Psicologia do ISMAT, Portimão, Portugal
[5] University of Michigan, Michigan, USA
{ocsmyth, mattpav}@umich.edu

Abstract. The impairment of basic cognitive functions such as attention and visual working memory can have a significant negative impact in our ability to adapt to the permanent changes in the environment. VR Serious Games are being used as a new tool for both assessment, stimulation and rehabilitation of such impaired functions. Even though the results of these novel applications seem to be promising, some of the assessments based in these solutions use indirect measures to evaluate attentional and mnesic performance (e.g. number of errors, task completion time). Gaze tracking (GT) can provide more accurate and direct indicators of these cognitive processes. On a sample of 46 non-clinical participants (33 Female; 71.7%), with an age average of 27.96 years old (SD = 11.92), ocular movements were recorded in two different comparative visual search tasks (CVSTs) that are an integrant part of the cognitive assessment protocol of the Systemic Lisbon Battery (SLB). Number of visits and total fixations differed based on the assessment with the Mini-mental state examination test (MMSE). These results highlight the possibility of combining both the data from the GT and the results of the "spot the differences" tasks in SLB, adding an unobtrusive and reliable solution for cognitive assessment in clinical and non-clinical settings.

Keywords: Gaze tracking · Eye movements · Attention · Memory · Serious games · Comparative search-task

© Springer International Publishing AG 2017
H.M. Fardoun et al. (Eds.): REHAB 2015, CCIS 665, pp. 26–34, 2017.
https://doi.org/10.1007/978-3-319-69694-2_3

1   Introduction

The intersection between neurological rehabilitation and Information and Communications Technologies (ICT) has been the subject of great interests in an expanding field of research. Within the neurological rehabilitation field, cognitive assessment and treatment usually targets different psychological dimensions such as attention, memory, and executive functions [1, 2], which aims to fix impairments while also teaching patients new skills to adapt in different environments.

Traditional paper-and-pencil assessments have been criticized for lacking complexity and efficiency when it comes to evaluating day-to-day tasks [3], leading research in ICT towards adapting more efficient means of rehabilitation. Though traditional methods do have their positive benefits, Virtual Reality Applications (VRAs) comprise an alternative way to assess performance, namely through: the ability to collect more cognitive information, safe engagement in recognizable settings, and task-oriented treatment [4, 5]. The premise of VRAs typically involves a dynamic, real world simulation that engages the user to interact in familiar scenarios and contexts [6]. Due to this, VRAs in cognitive assessment are able to target specific populations and evaluate the influence of various environmental stimuli on cognitive performance [7]. Additionally, game-like properties with positive feedback from VRAs can increase patient motivation [8] and directly translate into real world situations. Evidence shows that active engagement in rehabilitation plays a major role with regards to outcomes [9]. Both the Systemic Lisbon Battery (SLB) [10] and the Computer Assisted Rehabilitation Program-Virtual Reality (CARP-VR) [11] have demonstrated this capability and show promise for VRAs in the field of rehabilitation.

Along with VRAs, Gaze Tracking (GT) has shown the potential to improve assessment of cognitive functions for different disorders such as anxiety [12], addiction, [13] and even neurodegenerative diseases (e.g. Parkinson's, Alzheimer's, frontal-temporal dementia, etc.) [14]. Since human perception is very limited, only small amounts of information can be selected and processed at once [15]. GT allow estimating the orientation of eye in space and subsequently, to estimate user's point-of-regard, that can be thought as the position in a rendered content that the user is supposed to be viewing [16]. The analysis of the gaze behavior allows researchers and clinicians to evaluate ongoing cognitive processes [17]. In fact, eye-gaze movements allow us to better understand the underlying attentional processes [18].

VRAs and GT, though independently beneficial to the field of neurological rehabilitation, have also shown to be advantageous in combination for both assessment and treatment of cognitive impairments [19]. A pilot study was done in order to determine whether GT could be used to quantify engagement in real time within a VR task. Two main eye movement features were recorded: average eye movement speed and eye movement total displacement in a given time period. Results showed that mental engagement levels could be distinguished through patterns of eye movements in a multitude of games [20]. Another study wanted to compare social phenotypes between patients with Williams's syndrome (WS) and autism. Sixteen participants with WS and twenty-six participants with autism were recruited for the study. Ocular fixations and gaze time were recorded while each participant watched static images as well as movie extracts in order to evaluate socio-cognitive skills. Results showed that gaze behavior was linked to the way that socially relevant information was extracted [21].

Researchers in a different study looked at correlating aphasia with difficulty allocating attention, through GT. Twenty-six adults with aphasia and thirty-three control participants were given visual stimuli for auditory sentence comprehension and visual search tasks. Results showed that subjects with aphasia had more difficulty in allocating attention with each task. All together these results support assessment of allocating attention through the use of novel eye-tracking methods for individuals with and without aphasia. This method could potentially be used to assess responses of individuals following acquired brain injuries, and more closely look at secondary cognitive and physical impairments [22]. These studies give reason for further research in the growing field of GT. With this application, therapists could adjust in real time the virtual task to better suit the patient's needs and engagement levels.

Another study used GT to assess visual attention with children during serious games (SG). Heat maps, created based on entire time it took to complete each level, showed that individuals with weaker performances have higher fixation density than those who performed better. Despite these findings, VRAs in combination with GT are still in their early stages of research, and more studies should be conducted to ascertain stronger associations between gaze behavior and performance [23].

While evaluating cognitive functions and attention specifically, there are several known GT-based paradigms that demonstrate viable application [12, 15, 18]. One of these paradigms is the comparative visual search tasks (CVST) that assesses perceptual and attentional strategies. According to Galpin and Underwood [24] this experimental paradigm involves not only attention, but also a memory component as both are imperative to completing the task. Further support from Irwin [25] reiterates that the comparison of details between side-by-side images relies on the process of encoding into visual memory. Since attention is closely tied to memory, gaze behavior may mirror how observers coordinate visual mnemonic data and how attention is processed. In fact, this is advocated by Pomplun [26], claiming that the difference detection is served by a typified oculomotor behavior. In a recent study conducted by Rosa and colleagues [27], GT and SG were combined for assessing attentional and mnesic processes while performing CVST. In this study, three groups of participants were set based on Mini Mental State Examination (MMSE) normal range scores [28 (2 errors) vs 29 (1error) vs 30 (no errors)]. Participants with no errors on MMSE showed distinct gaze pattern characterized by lower fixation duration (TFD and less number of visits (NV), indicating a quicker visual information extraction of both images in comparison with both groups that presented errors on MMSE. Also the Time to task completion was longer in the groups with errors on MMSE than in the group with no errors. However, in this study the group with 2 errors consisted of only four participants, increasing variability and the sampling error. The present study is an extended version of that work as the sample size was increased and only two aggregate groups were compared (group with errors vs group with no errors), forming more balanced groups. Taking these prior studies into consideration, the aim of the present research was to assess gaze behavior as a function of cognitive ability in CVSTs. Our hypothesis is that gaze behavior, more specifically, TFD and NV between the two images may vary between groups with different cognitive abilities, validating the combined use of VR and GT for the assessment of attentional and mnesic processes.

2 Method

2.1 Participants

The sample of this study was 46 university students of the Universidade Lusófona de Humanidades e Tecnologias, in Lisbon. Of these, 71.7% were Female (n = 33). The average age of the sample was 27.96 years (SD = 11.92), ranging from 21 to 57 years old. Most participants were Portuguese (95.7%; n = 44) and reported normal medical history and no visual problems. The main exclusion criteria were: (i) MMSE [28] scores less than 28, and (ii) history of psychiatric disorders or drug addiction condition. All participants were well informed about the study and signed a written informed consent in accordance with APA's ethical principles of psychologists and code of conduct [29].

2.2 Stimuli

The stimuli consisted of two colorized paintings, one of Vincent van Gogh "The Night Café in the Place Lamartine in Arles" and the other one, a modified version of the "Son of Man" by René Magritte, both with a 1280 × 1024 resolution. Each image pairing was displayed side by side on a brown background (RGB: 68, 40, 22), separated by a distance of 2° of visual angle at the viewing distance of 60 cm. Each image subtended 11.81° × 7.63° of visual angle. Both image pairing depicted several objects with seven differences between them.

2.3 Measures

The protocol included a questionnaire on demographic details (gender, age, nationality) along with computer knowledge questions and the MMSE for screening general cognitive ability [28]. The MMSE was applied individually, which took circa 15 min. Two rectangular areas of interest (AoI) were manually drawn around each image as shown in Fig. 1.

TFD and NV were the proposed gaze metrics to assess attention and mnesic processes. Each visit was defined as the interval of time between the first fixation on the AoI and the next fixation outside the AoI.

2.4 Procedure and Apparatus

The experiment occurred in a single session, in a soundproof laboratory room with constant illumination (42 lx). Each participant signed a consent form and was seated at the distance of 60 cm from the eye tracker. After having successfully filled out the protocol, a 9-point calibration procedure was applied. The participants were instructed to search for the seven differences as quickly as possible and spot them at the right image through a mouse click. Two CVSTs, part of the SLB, were randomly presented.

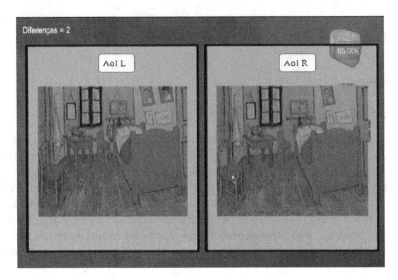

Fig. 1. Two manually drawn AoIs used for statistical analysis.

The SLB is a Unity 2.5-based (Unity Technologies[TM]) VRA consisting of a small town populated with digital robots (bots). The town is comprised of several buildings arranged in eight square blocks, along with a 2-room apartment mini-market and art gallery in its vicinity, where participants were able to visit [4] (see Fig. 2). The CVSTs embedded in SLB were displayed through in an Intel core2duo 6550 desktop computer, which was connected to a Tobii-T60 ET System (Tobii Technology AB, Sweden) and integrated into a 17″ TFT. Each CVST ended automatically when all the differences were correctly identified.

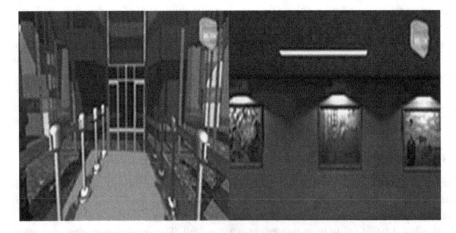

Fig. 2. The art gallery entrance in SLB (left) and the painting room where CVSTs were displayed (right).

The video signal from an Intel-based PC equipped with a GeForce GT 220 running SLB was captured through a VGA capture card installed in the eye tracker desktop. Eye movements were binocularly recorded at 60 Hz, with a spatial accuracy of 0.5° of visual angle, during whole the experiment. After both tasks were accomplished, participants were thanked, debriefed and finally dismissed.

3 Statistical Analysis and Results

Eye blinks, drifts, and outliers (±2 SD) were removed from raw gaze data and coded as missing values [15, 17, 30]. The percentage of missing values was lower than 1% and was randomly distributed across CVSTs. Two cognitive level groups were set apart based on MMSE, those who presented 1 or 2 errors (47.8%; $n = 22$) and those that had no errors on MMSE (52.2%; $n = 24$). A mixed factorial multivariate analysis of covariance (mixed-design MANCOVA) was performed to compare TFD and NV between the two cognitive level groups, using the participant's age as covariate. Age was included as covariate in our statistical model because is considered an important confounder of cognitive performance. Greenhouse-Geisser corrected degrees of freedom were used to report statistical significant levels. Bonferroni correction was applied for pairwise comparisons and statistical significance was set at $p < .05$

A 2 (AoI) × 2 (cognitive levels) MANCOVA revealed a main effect of the cognitive level on the composite variable that combined TFD and NV $\Lambda = 0.688$, F (2, 34) = 7.70, $p = .002$. A further univariate analysis showed a significant effect of the cognitive level on TFD F (1, 35) = 15.42, $p < .001$, $\eta_p^2 = .31$ and on NV, F (1, 35) = 11.48, $p = .002$, $\eta_p^2 = .25$, after the effect of age has been accounted for. With regard to TFD, the results showed that the group with no errors on MMSE had shorter TFD in both AoI ($M = 19.27$) than the group with errors on the MMSE ($M = 41.32$) as has shown in Fig. 3.

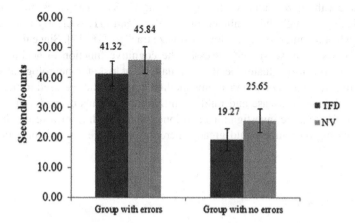

Fig. 3. Mean TFD (in seconds) and NV (number of visits) as a function of MMSE score after controlling for the effect of age. Error bars represent standard errors of the adjusted mean

4 Discussion

The findings of this study offer valuable insights into the relationship between high-order cognitive control processes and gaze behavior. The results showed that participants with the maximum score on MMSE display distinct gaze patterns characterized by a quicker detailed information processing (extraction) of both images (lower TFD) as compared to participants that presented errors on MMSE. This might be explained by low speed-loaded processes presented by the lower MMSE groups, which might have needed longer extraction time to reactivate memory representation [31]. With regards to NV, the groups that have presented errors on MMSE showed higher NV in comparison to the higher cognitive level group. In CSVTs, switching gaze usually occurs when a comparison is about to be made, and thus NV indicated how many eye movements were implicated in encoding before a comparison is elicited and the difference is noticed [32]. Our results support the idea that group with errors might have performed more visits between AoI due to a weak visual working memory usage. As the maintenance and processing of visual information decay quicker in lower MMSE groups, switching saccades between AoI are performed in order to rehearse the information [24]. More interesting was the fact that the reference image has shown more visits. This suggests that participants of this group might have used more the space between images to compare them simultaneously through peripheral attention, demonstrating a particular visual search strategy. This might be attributable to decrements in some cognitive abilities, especially in visual attention and visual memory. However, this study has some limitations that should be borne in mind when interpreting the findings. First, the level of fatigue was not controlled. Due to its interference with attentional processes [15], the level of fatigue should be assessed in future studies. Second, our sample was composed only by university students who have identical education and computer experience. In order to generalize our results to a broader population a heterogeneous sample should be gathered. Altogether, the results support the assumption that cognitive abilities (or the lack thereof), especially attention and memory, affect the gaze patterns when performing CVSTs. The assessment of cognitive functioning through the combined use of VRA and GT, is clearly advantageous, especially when it comes to current low-cost gaze trackers [16, 17]. Since the combined approach in this study sensitively assessed the cognitive function in healthy individuals, the potential to evaluate specific populations at risk for neurological diseases could be advantageous. For instance, this method could further be used to detect early stages of Alzheimer's disease and mild cognitive impairments or assess the disease's progression. With future investigations and longitudinal studies, measuring changes in visual processing over time could greatly increase predictive strength in neurological diseases.

References

1. Evans, J.: Cognitive rehabilitation: an integrative neuropsychological approach. Brain **126** (1), 261–262 (2003). doi:http://dx.doi.org/10.1093/brain/awg003
2. Gianutsos, R.: What is cognitive rehabilitation? J. Rehabil. **46**(3), 36–40 (1980)

3. Negut, A.: Cognitive assessment and rehabilitation in virtual reality: theoretical review and practical implications. Rom. J. Appl. Psychol. **16**, 1–7 (2014)
4. Alankus, G., Lazar, A., May, M., Kelleher, C.: Towards customizable games for stroke rehabilitation. In: Proceedings of the SIGCHI Conference on Human Factors in Computing Systems, Atlanta, USA, 10–15 April 2010, pp. 2113–2122. ACM Press, New York (2010)
5. Rego, P., Moreira, P.M., Reis, L.P.: Serious games for rehabilitation: a survey and a classification towards a taxonomy. In: Proceedings of the 5th Iberian Conference on Information Systems and Technologies (CISTI), Santiago de Compostela, Spain, 16–19 June 2010, pp. 1–6. IEEE press, New York (2010)
6. Parsey, C., Schmitter-Edgecombe, M.: Applications of technology in neuropsychological assessment. Clin. Neuropsychol. **27**, 10 (2013) doi:10.1080/13854046.2013.834971
7. Ortiz-Catalan, M., Nijenhuis, S., Ambrosch, K., Bovend'Eerdt, T., Koenig, S., Lange, B.: Virtual reality. In: Pons, J.L., Torricelli, D. (eds.) Emerging Therapies in Neurorehabilitation, Biosystems & Biorobotics, pp. 249–265. Springer, Heidelberg. doi:10.1007/978-3-642-38556-8_13
8. St-Jacques, J., Bouchard, S., Belanger, C.: Is virtual reality effective to motivate and raise interest in phobic children toward therapy? A clinical trial study of in vivo with in virtuo versus in vivo only treatment exposure. J. Clin. Psychiatry **71**(7), 924–931 (2010). doi:http://dx.doi.org/10.4088/JCP.08m04822blu
9. Burke, J., McNeill, M.D.J., Charles, D.K., Morrow, P.J., Crosbie, J.H., McDonough, M.: Optimising engagement for stroke rehabilitation using serious games. Vis. Comput. **25**(12), 1085–1099 (2009). doi:http://dx.doi.org/10.1007/s00371-009-0387-4
10. Gamito, P., et al.: Virtual kitchen test. Assessing frontal lobe functions in patients with alcohol dependence syndrome. Methods Inf. Med. **54**(2), 122–126 (2015). doi:http://dx.doi.org/10.3414/ME14-01-0003
11. Lam, Y.S., Man, D.W., Tam, S.F., Weiss, P.L.: Virtual reality training for stroke rehabilitation. Neuro Rehabil. **21**(3), 245–253 (2006)
12. Rosa, P.J., Gamito, P., Oliveira, J., Morais, D.: Attentional orienting to biologically fear-relevant stimuli: data from eye tracking using the continual alternation flicker paradigm. J. Eye Track. Vis. Emotion Cognit. **1**, 22–29 (2011)
13. Gamito, P., Oliveira, J., Baptista, A., Morais, D., Lopes, P., Rosa, P., Santos, N., Brito, R.: Eliciting nicotine craving with virtual smoking cues. Cyberpsychol. Behav. Soc. Netw. **17**(8), 556–561 (2014). doi:http://dx.doi.org/10.1089/cyber.2013.0329
14. Cipresso, P., Serino, S., Gaggioli, A., Albani, G., Riva, G.: Contactless bio-behavioral technologies for virtual reality. Stud. Health Technol. Inform. **191**, 149–153 (2013)
15. Rosa, P.J., Esteves, F., Arriaga, P.: Effects of fear-relevant stimuli on attention: integrating gaze data with subliminal exposure. In: Proceedings of the Medical Measurements and Applications (MeMeA), Lisbon, Portugal, June 12–14, pp. 8–14. doi:10.1109/MeMeA2014.6860021
16. Rosa, P.J.: What do your eyes say? Bridging eye movements to consumer behavior. Int. J. Psychol. Res. **8**(2), 91–104 (2015)
17. Rosa, P.J., Esteves, F., Arriaga, P.: Beyond traditional clinical measurements for screening fears and phobias. IEEE Trans. Instrum. Measur. **64**(12), 3396–3404 (2015). doi:http://dx.doi.org/10.1109/TIM.2015.2450292
18. Banovic, M., Chrysochou, P., Grunert, K., Rosa, P.J., Gamito, P.: The effect of fat content on visual attention and choice of red meat and differences across gender. Food Qual. Prefer. **52**, 42–51 (2016). doi:http://dx.doi.org/10.1016/j.foodqual.2016.03.017
19. Mele, M., Federici, S.: A psychotechnological review on eye-tracking systems: towards user experience. Disabil. Rehabil. Assist. Technol. **7**(4), 261–281 (2012). doi:http://dx.doi.org/10.3109/17483107.2011.635326

20. Vidal, M., Turner, J., Bulling, A., Gellersen, H.: Wearable eye tracking for mental health monitoring. Comput. Commun. **35**(11), 1306–1311 (2012). http://dx.doi.org/10.1016/j.comcom.2011.11.002

21. Riby, D., Hancock, P.J.: Looking at movies and cartoons: eye-tracking evidence from Williams's syndrome and autism. J. Intellect. Disabil. Res. **53**(2), 169–181. doi:http://dx.doi.org/10.1111/j.1365-2788.2008.01142.x

22. Deng, S., Kirkby, J., Chang, J., Zhang, J.: Multimodality with eye tracking and haptics: a new horizon for serious games? Int. J. Serious Games **1**(4), 17–33 (2014)

23. Frutos-Pascual, M., Garcia-Zapirain, B.: Assessing visual attention using eye tracking sensors in intelligent cognitive therapies based on serious games. Sensors **15**(5), 11092 (2015). doi:10.3390/s150511092

24. Galpin, A.J., Underwood, G.: Eye movements during search and detection in comparative visual search. Percept. Psychophys. **67**(8), 1313–1331 (2005)

25. Irwin, D.E., Zelinsky, G.J.: Eye movements and scene perception: memory for things observed. Percept. Psychophys. **64**(6), 882–895 (2002)

26. Pomplun, M., Sichelschmidt, L., Wagner, K., Clermont, T., Rickheit, G., Ritter, H.: Comparative visual search: a difference that makes a difference. Cognit. Sci. **25**(1), 3–36 (2001). doi:http://dx.doi.org/10.1207/s15516709cog2501_2

27. Rosa, P.J., Gamito, P., Oliveira, J., Morais, D., Pavlovic, M., Smyth, O.: Show me your eyes! The combined use of eye tracking and virtual reality applications for cognitive assessment. In: Proceedings of the 3rd 2015 Workshop on ICTs for Improving Patients Rehabilitation Research Techniques, Lisbon, Portugal, 1-2 October 2015, pp. 135–138. ACM Press, New York (2015). doi:10.1145/2838944.2838977

28. Folstein, M., Folstein, S., McHugh, P.: Mini-mental state a practical method for grading the cognitive state of patients for the clinician. J. Psychiatr. Res. **12**(3), 189–198 (1975)

29. American Psychological Association. Ethical principles of psychologists and code of conduct. http://apa.org/ethics/code/index.aspx. Accessed 11 Jan 2016

30. Rosa, P.J., Gamito, P., Oliveira, J., Morais, D., Pavlovic, M., Smyth, O.: Uso de eye tracking em realidade virtual não imersiva para avaliação cognitiva. Psicologia Saúde Doenças **17**(1), 23–31 (2016)

31. Gottlob, L.R.: Aging and comparative search for feature differences. Aging Neuropsychol. Cognit. **13**(3-4) 435–457 (2006). doi:http://dx.doi.org/10.1080/138255890969564

32. Mcafoose, J., Baune, B.T.: Exploring visual-spatial working memory: a critical review of concepts and models. Neuropsychol. Rev. **19**(1), 130–142 (2009). doi:http://dx.doi.org/10.1007/s11065-008-9063-0

Pressure Data and Multi-material Approach to Design Prosthesis

Claudio Comotti, Daniele Regazzoni, Caterina Rizzi$^{(\boxtimes)}$, and Andrea Vitali

Department of Management, Information and Production Engineering,
University of Bergamo, Bergamo, Italy
{claudio.comotti,daniele.regazzoni,caterina.rizzi,
andrea.vitali1}@unibg.it

Abstract. This paper concerns the design and manufacture of medical devices, such as lower limb prosthesis, integrating low cost industrial technologies. In particular, it focuses the attention on the custom-fit component of a lower limb prosthesis, i.e., the socket, that is the interface with the residual limb. The considered process starts from the 3D reconstruction of patients' limb and ends with the manufacture of the socket with a 3D printer using a multi-material approach. The process counts three steps: 3D modeling, testing (both experimental and numerical) and manufacturing. For each step adopted solutions and tools are described. Finally, conclusions are drawn mainly concerning the challenge of multi-material 3D printing of the socket.

Keywords: 3D printing · Socket Modelling Assistant · Lower limb prosthesis

1 Introduction

During last years, many breakthrough ICT technologies are launched on the market but not all the industrial sectors are ready to quickly adopt them. Leap Motion, Oculus Rift and MS Kinect are only a few of these devices that allow interacting with the virtual prototype in an unconventional and revolutionary way [1, 2]. Nowadays, many fields exploit reverse engineering methods since they guarantee the reconstruction and the visualization of a real object. For this reason, it is possible to find on the market many different applications [3], such as dental scanning for medical purposes [4] or body scanning to best fit a dress on the customer [5–7]. Other applications adopt ICTs in daily process allowing the interaction with virtual models. Actually, in the medical field it is required to severely assess the reliability and robustness of any technical novelties, either for diagnostic purpose or for treatment. Two main leverages that can shorten the introduction of new technical solutions in the medical field are: (i) a high level of automation in the process, so that any system can perform most of the work without human intervention and (ii) the adoption of high-performing low-cost devices derived from other application sectors (e.g., entertainment or video gaming industry). A low cost philosophy allows having a large potential diffusion on the market. According to this approach, this research work presents a full-virtual method to model, test and manufacture lower limb prosthesis that in a near future will hopefully take place the traditional empirical

H.M. Fardoun et al. (Eds.): REHAB 2015, CCIS 665, pp. 35–45, 2017.
https://doi.org/10.1007/978-3-319-69694-2_4

method. Nowadays, prosthetic CAD systems already exist, but our aim has been to develop a design framework that permits to automate some steps of the product development process and embed prosthetists' knowledge and easily affordable also by small orthopedic labs. There are several phases in which HW and SW solutions may be applied. For instance, manual measurement of anthropometric data can be replaced by diagnostic image processing or by 3D scanning to create a 3D model of the anatomical district. Such model can be virtually edited to create the appropriate functional shape according to embedded knowledge. Moreover, some test and validation procedures can be performed on the virtual model before dealing with real components, thus, anticipating potential failures and early fixing otherwise costly issues. At last, manufacturing may rely on the virtual model and 3D printing technology can be profitably used, not only to shorten production times but also to create high performance customized solutions for each patient.

In this paper, firstly, the traditional process to manufacture lower limb prosthesis is introduced; then, the proposed methods and tools to accomplish the innovative way to design, test and manufacturing of the prosthesis are described. Finally, conclusions are drawn mainly concerning the challenge of multi-material 3D printing of the socket.

The paper constitutes an extension of the research work presented by V&K Group at the REHAB 2015: 3rd workshop on ICTs for improving Patients Rehabilitation Research Techniques [8].

2   Lower Limb Traditional Manufacturing Process

The socket is the most critical component for both transfemoral and transtibial prostheses. It is manufactured from a positive chalk cast of the residual limb. The cast can be manufactured following a full handmade procedure or partially based on CAD/CAM systems [9]. During traditional manufacturing process, the technician continuously uses hands to achieve the most functional and comfortable socket shape. At first, s/he does an evaluation of the amputee and creates a negative cast manipulating by hands plaster patches directly on patient's residual limb. Then, orthopedic technician builds the positive model (Fig. 1a) by adding and removing chalk in specific zones according to residuum size and patient's features (e.g., muscles tonicity). Three main manual operations are performed: initial plaster circumference reduction, identification and marking of critical zones, and critical zones manipulation. The first operation consists in a reduction of positive plaster cast according to residual limb conditions. For example, the socket must be more fitting for young or recently amputated patients, while for elderly patients it needs to be a bit loose to allow an easier gait or rehabilitation activities. In the second step the technician marks with a pencil on the positive cast the areas that have to be modified. The third step consists in adding or removing materials in highlighted critical zones (Fig. 1b). We identified these critical zones, which are different for transtibial and transfemoral amputees, and can be classified as:

- Load zones where there are no bony protuberances or tendons. In this case the plaster has to be removed in order to have a self-supporting tighter socket.

- Off-load zones where there are bony protuberances or tendons. In this case the technician adds material on the positive plaster cast since in that zones the socket does not have to press the limb and be slightly loose.

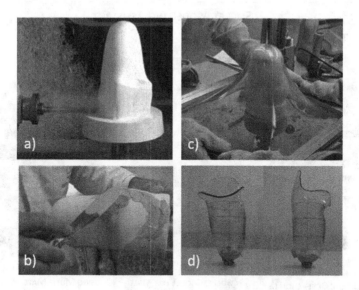

Fig. 1. Some of the traditional steps of the socket manufacturing process.

After this, a thermoformed check socket (Fig. 1d) is manufactured directly on the modified positive model and tested on the patient by heating and displacing a plastic layer on the reproduction of the residual limb (Fig. 1c). Other necessary modifications are sketched on the positive model to realize a more comfortable and well-fitting final socket. Finally, the definitive socket is realized and all the prosthesis components are assembled for the final static set-up. Summarizing, the socket is manufactured following a hand-made procedure and the final shape heavily depends on the prosthetist's skills and experience. Even if the socket has been designed starting from patient's features, the socket design does not take in consideration several aspects relative to the material hardness that usually creates fatigue and sickness to the amputees during gait along both load and off-load zones. This issue could be approached by exploiting 3D printing technology.

3   Proposed Method

The proposed method is centered on the virtual representation of the patient's residual limb. Even if the virtual process is highly integrated and the data flow is as fluid as possible, three main phases can be identified as modeling, test and manufacturing of socket. As shown in Fig. 2, firstly the technician uses Socket Modelling Assistant (SMA) to model the initial socket shape. Then, a pressure analysis is executed until the best socket shape has been achieved. After that, STL files are exported according to selected materials for load zones and the rest of socket. Finally, a multi-material 3D printer is used to build the socket.

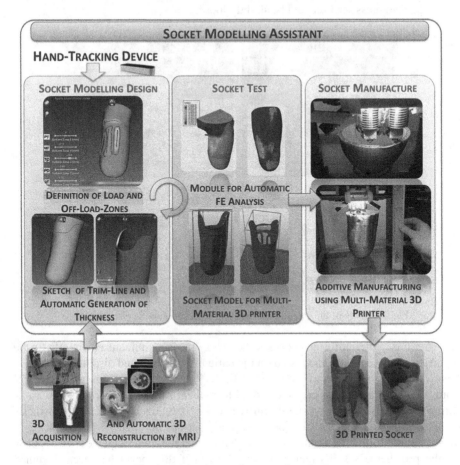

Fig. 2. Main phases of proposed method.

3.1   Socket Design

In the last decade, our research group has been developing an ad-hoc knowledge-guided CAD system, which allows the prosthetist to design the socket of both transtibial and transfemoral prosthesis relying on the digital model of the residual limb (Fig. 2) [10]. SMA emulates all phases of the socket development process starting from the digital model of the residual limb acquired either by Magnetic Resonance Imaging (MRI) [11] or using a low cost RGB-D depth sensor. The prosthetist is guided step-by-step by the system that applies in automatic or semi-automatic way the rules and the modelling procedures. It embeds a set of design rules and procedures (e.g., where and how to modify the socket shape) and makes available a set of interactive virtual tools to manipulate the socket shape according to traditional procedures. Furthermore, we have developed a module, which exploits hand-tracking devices (e.g., Leap Motion device) in order to emulate the design operation as traditionally made by orthopedic technicians who use their hands to shape the socket [2].

SMA includes a set of tools as follows:

- *Module for patient data acquisition* to insert anthropometric data and 3D model of bones and residual limb.
- *Circumferences scaling tool* to scale the initial model like the orthopedic technician does in the traditional process to reduce the volume. In particular, the technician first identifies on the plaster cast the same reference circumferences previously measured on the patient's residual limb, and then starts to file harmoniously the plaster until these circumferences are reduced of the desired percentages. Through a set of cross section planes, the user can decide the reduction percentage in correspondence of each of them.
- *Marker tool* to mark on the surface of the virtual residual limb both off-load and load zones with different colors.
- *Deformation tool* to emulate the operation of adding/removing chalk during traditional process on the previously colored zones. If the zone is an off-load zone the mesh of the marked area is pushed inside of a certain quantity according to patient's characteristics, specifically the residuum tonicity; otherwise if it is a load zone the mesh inside the contour is pushed outside.
- *Definition of socket lower part* that represents an important operation to obtain a no-pain socket.
- *Sculpt tool* to interactively manipulate the shape of the socket. The operations allowed on the socket mesh are in/deflate, smoothing and flattening.
- *Trim-line tool* to define in a semi-automatic mode the border line of the socket on the base of templates defined according to orthopedic knowledge.

Beyond the technical challenge of creating such a complex ICT tool, the relevance of this part is mainly due to the inner connection it has with the medical application. The module has been built exploiting orthopedic knowledge extracted from physicians' interviews and best cases, coded and embedded into the system. Moreover, the real applicative condition in a prosthetic lab has been kept in high consideration when designing the process and the user's interface. This should ease the transition to a digital way of designing the socket.

3.2 Socket Test and Experimentation

Socket shape must be tested and optimized and for this reason we approached the problem by means of two methods, experimental and numerical, and parameter to evaluate patient pain is the contact pressure at the interface between the internal surface of the socket and the skin of the residual limb. The underline idea is to make available a design framework that permits to automatically analyze the pressure at the interface socket-residual limb and avoid the pressure acquisition, on the base of pressure data coming out from the numerical simulation. Therefore, through the comparison of experimental and numerical distribution of pressure, we assessed a simulation.

We first executed an experimental approach that is also useful to validate the numerical one. To this end, the Tekscan F-Socket system able to map the distribution of pressure acting on the sensors has been considered. It is composed by six sensors 9811E, two VersaTek Cuffs and a VersaTek Port Hub. The sensors have a resistive core with silver connections comprised between two thin plastic layers. Sensitive areas, called *sensels*, are displaced according to a matrix pattern of 6 × 16 cells. This system performs a direct measure of pressure and guarantees a good compromise between data quality and acquired signal [12]. Known issues concerning signal drift, dependence on load frequency and on curvature, affect this type of sensors. The main problem we faced was the signal drift, because we do not use high curvatures and the load frequency is not relevant. Some tests have been performed to this aim and, adopting some precautions, signal drift can be dramatically reduced. How to dispose sensors over the residual limb (Fig. 3) required particular attention due to residual limb shape, adhesion of sensors and soft tissue. After some tests (e.g., sensors fixed on the socket, sensors positioned in different directions), we chose to displace sensors vertically on the patient's skin using a thin plastic film to improve their fixing. This reduces the formation of creases on the sensor surface and permits to position sensors in critical zones on the residual limb and avoid possible shifting due to the donning.

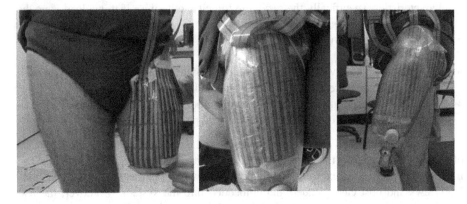

Fig. 3. Pressure sensors displacement on the residual limb of a transfemoral amputee patient

We executed some tests in static position by loading 50% and 100% of patient weight on the artificial leg and also in dynamic condition by acquiring data during some gait cycles. From acquired data it was possible to extract the distribution of pressure on the residual limb and visualize it in a three dimensional environment using an ad-hoc developed module. The application visualizes the 3D model of the residual limb, which is acquired with 3D scanning previously described. The 3D model is imported in OBJ format in which the vertex color data has been added with the Skanect exporting module [13]. The 3D scanning of the residual limb with sensors applied (Fig. 4a) permits the 3D mapping of the sensors in the correct position by using the visualization of the 3D colored model. The use of the application is based on two main phases: sensors mapping and data analysis. Figure 4b shows the outcome where the pressure values are mapped on the residual limb geometry acquired with MS Kinect. Even if numerical test has been carried out to assess the numerical approach, it can be independently used to validate any physical socket already realized and used by patients and identify design mistakes.

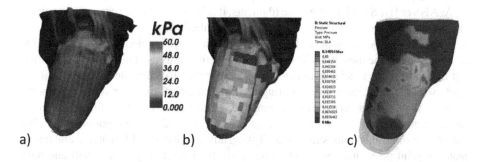

Fig. 4. (a) 3D model acquired by MS Kinect of a residual limb with pressure sensors, Pressure map obtain with (b) experimental data and (c) FE simulation between residual limb and socket.

Regarding the numerical approach, the main challenge has been to implement an automatic procedure to provide the medical staff with Finite Element simulation results without the intervention of a simulation expert. Moreover, the outcome of simulation highlights eventual pressure peaks or other issues that can be passed to SMA in order to be automatically fixed. The numerical simulation required the definition of a number of parameters guiding the process and of simulations rules related to: geometric model, mesh, material characterization, analysis steps, and boundary conditions. They have been derived from an extensive analysis of the state of the art, from the experience acquired in previous research activities, and by balancing accuracy of results and computational costs. Details about the SW tools, the 3D model definition and the simulation parameters can be found in [14–16]. As said simulation results can be handled in background so that no expert is required, by the way to control the shape change operated by SMA a graphical representation of the pressure distribution can be shown (Fig. 4c).

Once the iterations among the design and test phases is completed, i.e. when the patient's load does not create critical pressure conditions, the output can be generated in order to proceed with the socket manufacture. SMA automatically exports two STL files, corresponding to the load and off-load zones and, thus, the different material to be used for the manufacturing. At the moment, the simulation outcomes are comparable to the real distribution of the pressure on the residual limb.

3.3 Socket Manufacture

Additive manufacturing allows creating real models, which are already usable for testing and simulation. In the last years the development of this application field was very quick. New 3D printing machines and materials have been introduced in the global market as well many challenges in a lot of field such as industrial, design, medical, scientific or daily scopes [17]. The range of materials that is possible to use in 3D printing application is very large and constantly growing. Plastic materials, bio-materials, steel, ceramic, clay are just a few that can be printed nowadays. FDM (Fuse Deposition Modeling) by

Stratasys [18] and FFF (Fused Filament Fabrication) by RepRap [19] are 3D printing methods that consist in the extrusion of fused material on the printing plane by layers [20]. This process is used especially with plastic filaments of different composition like PLA, ABS or HIPS [21]. Using these filaments, it is important to take care to the warping caused by the fusion and the fast cooling during the deposition process. PLA (Poly lactic acid or poly lactide) is biodegradable thermoplastic polyester derived from renewable resources and is the most used. These are the main materials used in 3D plastic printing, but there are some special filaments for particular uses like flexible filaments that are made with a rubber material permitting great deformation, or water soluble filaments useful to realize supports to be easily removed. This variety of printing filaments allows the integration of multiple materials in the same object: in this way it is possible to realize object with different composition areas. Taking advantage of flexible material and multi-material print possibility, new 3D printer permits to create object with soft and hard parts. Another important parameter is the infill density and shape. The internal structure conferred to the printed component contributes substantially to confer it rigidity and deformability. The internal grid can follow a twisted rectangular shape, honeycomb or round path (Fig. 5).

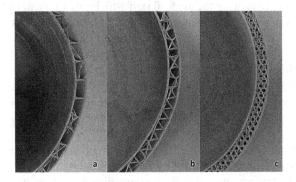

Fig. 5. Several infill modes: (a) 5% (b) 10% (c) 20%

An interesting study [22] on the relation between infill properties and functional features of the object highlights the great potential of additive manufacturing. In that research work, authors identify classes of standard infill cells that allow different behaviors only analyzing Young modulus and Poisson coefficient. The relationship between internal grid shape and the features of the part is very strong: the internal structure is manually created in relation to the stiffness required by the component. The transformation from 3D model to 3D geometry ready to be printed is the base to obtain multi-material object. The different characteristics of the volumes, obtained by varying the density through the fill and the different materials, is the most important element that gives the socket the local mechanical characteristics necessary to find a good compromise between comfort and structural strength. All these simulations and methods were applied to a case study with a patient with a lower limb prosthesis. This patient is a middle age man without the left leg and he uses a transtibial prosthesis. The study focused on the creation of an adaptive socket based on the residual limb geometry of the patient. In this application the socket composition was determined in relation to load and off-load areas of the socket: external coating is made with hard material, internal surface is composed by different areas made of soft material for off-load zone and hard material for load zone. Off-load zones have not to support excessive loads, but should only ensure structural strength and comfort to the patient. Load zones, conversely, must ensure a good compromise between mechanical resistance and comfort: they have to support all the height of the person and at the same time guarantee a full painless contact. In this paper all issues about infill, materials and comfort were engaged and solved with solutions with different compositions of materials.

The socket was realized with the 3D printer "Leonardo 300 Cube" by Meccatronicore (Fig. 6). This printer permits the multi-material printing with two different extruders. The application target is to obtain a perfect socket based on the residual limb geometry that guarantees a comfortable fit and an ideal matching. This approach avoids the patient to do several orthopedic visits to correct socket shape.

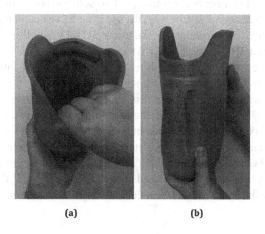

Fig. 6. Interior (a) and exterior (b) of the 3D printed socket.

4   Conclusions

Emerging technologies such a low-cost 3D scanners or 3D printing have a potential huge impact in several applications in which real life habits or custom fit products are involved. By the way, in some domains the level of robustness and required reliability are much higher than the level provided by emerging technologies and this slows down the innovation process. It also happens frequently that new technological solutions require an expert of the domain in which the technology has been developed and this is conflicting with the low-cost approach. The research work shown in this paper, beyond the technical complexity of the engineering solutions developed, is focused on the real usability of the final solutions for a non-technical operator. The underlying approach consists on one hand in embedding into the system all the routine and standard pieces of knowledge, rules and parameters; on the other hand, the intervention of the operator is asked whenever a decision making step is required. According to this approach, the design, test and manufacture of lower limb prosthetic socket has been radically changed. The traditional process is not computer aided and strictly relies on the manual ability of the prosthetist. The method and the tools proposed, on the contrary, are aimed at creating a 3D virtual representation of the residual limb, so that each design action can be performed on the digital model of the product rather than on a physical mock-up. The test can be performed without involving the patient and adopting his/her avatar to perform donning, static loading and gait simulations. The feasibility of each of these phases has been already investigated in previous works and what was still missing is a complete process going from patient data acquisition to prosthesis manufacture. The first two phases of the proposed procedure, i.e. socket design and socket test, have been developed trying to virtually replicate the manual process. Pressure acquisition was necessary to assess and optimize the numerical simulation, but only in a preliminary phase. The final procedure does not require a pressure acquisition on the patient. In the last phase, the production process consists in laminating a sheet of plastic polymer and to reinforce it with carbon fiber or other tissues. This solution is excellent for mechanical resistance and it is widespread. By the way, the use of additive manufacturing techniques opens at least two great opportunities: (i) the use of 3D internal filling of the socket wall to balance resistance and lightweight and (ii) the combined use of materials with different mechanical properties (e.g., different stiffness) to create hard and soft parts in specific zones of a one-piece socket. There is still some open issues on the use of 3D printed materials for daily used sockets. Material is hard to be characterized and, thus, to be approved as safe and reliable. However, the huge diffusion and research carried out in 3D printers will probably fix these issues in a short term and allow to produce robust, lightweight and reliable socket in a near future. Future developments will concern the investigation of all benefits that could offer other additive manufacturing methods, other materials and the optimization of infill and shape. The study of all these properties is finalized to create a final socket that is usable in all days' activities and not only a check socket.

References

1. Colombo, G., Regazzoni, D., Rizzi, C.: Ergonomic design through virtual humans. Comput. Aided Des. Appl. **10**(5), 745–755 (2013). doi:10.3722/cadaps.2013.745-755
2. Colombo, G., Facoetti, G., Rizzi, C., Vitali, A.: Low cost hand-tracking devices to design customized medical devices. In: Shumaker, R., Lackey, S. (eds.) VAMR 2015. LNCS, vol. 9179, pp. 351–360. Springer, Cham (2015). doi:10.1007/978-3-319-21067-4_36
3. Wasenmüller, O., Peters, J.C., Golyanik, V., Stricker, D.: Precise and automatic anthropometric measurement extraction using template registration. In: 6th International Conference on 3D Body Scanning Technologies, Lugano (2015). doi:10.15221/15.155
4. Salmi, M.: Medical applications of additive manufacturing in surgery and dental care. Ph.D. thesis, Aalto University, Helsinki (2013)
5. Wang, C.C.L.: CAD tools in fashion/garment design. Comput. Aided Des. Appl. **1**(1–4), 53–62 (2004). doi:10.1080/16864360.2004.10738243
6. Wang, C.H.; Chiang, Y.C., Wang, M.J.: Evaluation of an augmented reality embedded on-line shopping system. In: 6th International Conference on Applied Human Factors and Ergonomics, vol. 3, pp. 5624–5630. doi:10.1016/j.promfg.2015.07.766

7. Fontana, M., Rizzi, C., Cugini, U.: A CAD-oriented cloth simulation system with stable and efficient ODE solution. Comput. Graph. (Pergamon). **30**(3), 391–407 (2006). doi:10.1016/j.cag.2006.02.002
8. Comotti, C., Regazzoni, D., Rizzi, C., Vitali, A.: Multi-material design and 3D printing method of lower limb prosthetic sockets. In: Proceedings of the 3rd 2015 Workshop on ICTs for improving Patients Rehabilitation Research Techniques, pp. 42–45. ACM (2015). doi:10.1145/2838944.2838955
9. Singh, U.: Role of cad-cam technology in prosthetics and orthotics. In: Essentials of Prosthetics and Orthotics, p. 86 (2013)
10. Buzzi, M., Colombo, G., Facoetti, G., Gabbiadini, S., Rizzi, C.: 3D modelling and knowledge: tools to automate prosthesis development process. Int. J. Interact. Des. Manuf. **6**, 41–53 (2012). doi:10.1007/s12008-011-0137-5
11. Colombo, G., Facoetti, G., Rizzi, C., Vitali, A., Zanello, A.: Automatic 3D reconstruction of transfemoral residual limb from MRI images. In: Duffy, V.G. (ed.) DHM 2013. LNCS, vol. 8026, pp. 324–332. Springer, Heidelberg (2013). doi:10.1007/978-3-642-39182-8_38
12. Polliack, A.A., Sieh, R.C., Craig, D.D., Landsberger, S., McNeil, D.R., Ayyappa, E.: Scientific validation of two commercial pressure sensor systems for prosthetic socket fit. Prosthet. Orthot. Int. **24**(1), 63–73 (2000). doi:10.1080/03093640008726523
13. Skanect software. http://skanect.occipital.com/
14. Sengeh, D., Herr, H.: A variable-impedance prosthetic socket for a transtibial amputee designed from magnetic resonance imaging data. J. Prosthet. Orthotics **25**(3), 129–137 (2013). doi:10.1097/JPO.0b013e31829be19c
15. Lee, W.C., Zhang, M., Mak, A.F.: Regional differences in pain threshold and tolerance of the transtibial residual limb: including the effects of age and interface material. Arch. Phys. Med. Rehabil. **86**(4), 641–649 (2005)
16. Dumbleton, T., Buis, A.W.P., Mcfadyen, A., Mchugh, B.F., Mckay, G., Murray, K.D., Sexton, S.: Dynamic interface pressure distributions of two transtibial prosthetic socket concepts. J. Rehabil. Res. Dev. **46**(3), 405–415 (2009)
17. Aherwar, A., Singh, A., Patnaik, A.: A review paper on rapid prototyping and rapid tooling techniques for fabrication of prosthetic socket, pp. 345–353 (2014)
18. FDM by Stratasys. http://www.stratasys.com/3d-printers/technologies/fdm-technology
19. FFF by RepRap. http://reprap.org/wiki/Fused_filament_fabrication
20. Shi, Z., Peng, Y., Wei, W.: Recent advance on fused deposition modeling. Recent Patents Mech. Eng. **7**(2), 122–130 (2014). doi:10.2174/2212797607666140515231742
21. Rodriguez, J., Thomas, J.P., Renaud, J.E.: Mechanical behavior of acrylonitrile butadiene styrene (abs) fused deposition materials. Experimental investigation. Rapid Prototyping J. **7**(3), 148–158 (2001). doi:10.1108/13552540110395547
22. Schumacher, C., Bickel, B., Rys, J., Marschner, S., Daraio, C., Gross, M.: Microstructures to control elasticity in 3D printing. ACM Trans. Graph. **34**(4), Article 136 (2015). doi:10.1145/2766926

An Auditory Feedback Based System for Treating Autism Spectrum Disorder

Massimo Magrini[1(✉)], Andrea Carboni[1], Ovidio Salvetti[1],
and Olivia Curzio[2]

[1] ISTI – CNR, Pisa, Italy
{massimo.magrini,andrea.carboni,
ovidio.salvetti}@isti.cnr.it
[2] IFC – CNR, Pisa, Italy
oliviac@ifc.cnr.it

Abstract. A system for real-time gesture tracking is presented, used in active well-being self-assessment activities and in particular applied to medical coaching and music-therapy. The system is composed of a gestural interface and a computer running own (custom) developed software. During the test sessions a person freely moves his body inside a specifically designed room. The algorithms detect and extrapolate features from the human figure, such us spatial position, arms and legs angles, etc. An operator can link these features to sounds synthesized in real time, following a predefined schema. The augmented interaction with the environment helps to improve the contact with reality in subjects having autism spectrum disorders (ASD). The system has been tested on a set of young subjects and a team of psychologists has analyzed the results of this experimentation. Moreover, we developed a home version of the system, to be used without any operators, in order to maintain the obtained benefits. This paper is an extended version of the paper presented at REHAB 2015 [1].

Keywords: Human-computer interaction · Biofeedback · Autism

1 Introduction

In recent years specific activity has been carried out for developing sensor-based interactive systems capable to help the treatment of learning difficulties and disabilities in children [2, 3]. These systems generally consist of sensors connected to a computer, programmed with special software that reacts to the sensor data with multimedia stimuli. The general philosophy of these systems is based on the idea that even profoundly physically or learning impaired individuals can become expressive and communicative using music and sound [4]. The sense of control which these systems provide can be a powerful motivator for subjects with limited interaction with reality.

While a great part of systems, like SoundBeam (www.soundbeam.co.uk), totally rely on ultrasonic sensors, our approach is mostly based on real-time video processing techniques; moreover, our solution makes also it possible to easily use additional sets of sensors (e.g., infrared or ultrasonic) in the same scene. The use of video-processing techniques adds more parameters suitable to localize exactly and detail all the human

© Springer International Publishing AG 2017
H.M. Fardoun et al. (Eds.): REHAB 2015, CCIS 665, pp. 46–58, 2017.
https://doi.org/10.1007/978-3-319-69694-2_5

gestures we want detect and recognize. By using a custom software interface, the operator can link the extracted video features to sounds synthesized in real time, following a predefined schema.

The developed system has been experimented in a test campaign on a set of young patients affected by Low-Functioning Autism (autism spectrum disorder, ASD), in order to provide a personal increased interaction over the operational environment and to reduce pathological isolation [5]. Results were very positive and encouraging, as confirmed by both clinical psychologist and parents of the kids. In particular, the therapists reported a positive outcome from the assisted coaching therapies. Indeed, this positive evolution was crucial to improve the motivation and curiosity for a full communication interaction in the external environment, thus affecting subjects' well-being.

In order to maintain the obtained benefits, we developed a simplified version of the system, based on Kinect, to be used at home by the parents and children. The present project program trains parents of children with autistic spectrum disorders using the DIR/Floortime model of Stanley Greenspan MD. Parents were encouraged to deliver 15 h per week of 1:1 interaction. Pilot studies [6, 7] suggested that this kind of models have potential to be a cost-effective intervention for young children with autism.

2 Autism

ASD is a neurodevelopmental disorder characterized by impaired social interaction and communication. It is a pervasive developmental disorder, characterized by a triad of impairments: social communication problems, difficulties with reciprocal social inter-actions, and unusual patterns of repetitive behavior [8]. Leo Kanner, a child psychiatrist [8], described it for the first time in 1943. An exhaustive description of this disorder in medical terms is beyond the scope of this paper.

Unfortunately, no medications can cure autism or treat its core symptoms, but rather can help some people affected feel better. A large part of the interventions focuses on behavioral approaches, of which the best known is the ABA (Applied Behavior Analysis) method [10], based on repetitive patterns and reinforcements. Other approaches follow instead the Developmental Individual Difference Relationship (DIR) model [11]. DIR acts at various levels of involvement, attempting a containing action against the central symptoms of autism according to the following guidelines: (1) involvement against isolation (2) communication and flexibility versus rigidity and persistence (3) gestures against stereotypies and aggressive behaviors. In the design of our system we were inspired, even not strictly, by the DIR model.

3 The System

The system was developed in two different steps, using different technologies. The first version is based over video capture and processing, where all the body recognition routines are software-based. This system needed a controlled environment and the presence of a technician during each session. The second version relies on the use of

Kinect v2, which solved some of the problems of the previous version. This version allows the tracking of full body movements in 3D space, has the peculiarity of being designed to be installed in the user's home, and provides an intuitive interface, to be easily used by the children's families.

3.1 Camera Based Version

The first version of the system has been based on real-time video processing. The software has been developed in C++ on an Apple Macintosh computer running the latest version of Mac OS X. A video camera is connected through a Firewire digitizer, the Imaging Source DFG1394, a very fast digitizer that allows a latency of only one frame in the video processing path. As output audio card we use the Macintosh internal one, sufficient for our purposes. A couple of TASCAM amplified loudspeakers completes the basic system.

We used the Mac OS platform for its reliability in real time multimedia applications, thanks to its very robust frameworks: Core Audio and Core Image libraries permit very fast elaboration without glitches and underruns.

Finally, the system is installed in a special empty room, with most of the surfaces (walls, floor) covered by wood. The goal is to build a warm space which, in some way, recalls the prenatal ambient. All system parts, such as cables, plugs, and so on are carefully hidden as they could be potential elements of distraction. The ambient light is gentle and indirect, thus avoiding shadows that could also affect the precision of motion detection. Nevertheless, large changes in the environment light may affect the system's setup, so that the software needs some recalibration.

System Architecture. The implemented system (Fig. 1) is organized in several specialized coordinated modules. The core of the software is composed by the Sequence grabber, which manages the stream of video frames coming from the video digitizer, the Video processor, which performs realtime image elaborations, the Skeleton reconstructor, which analyses the frames and extrapolates gesture parameters, the Data mapper, responsible for transforming the detected gesture parameters into sounds parameters and finally the Sound synthesizer.

The biggest problem regarding the gesture control of sounds is latency, which is the delay between the gesture and the correspondent effect on the generated sound.

Our approach guarantees the minimum latency for the adopted frame rate, which is 40 ms at 25 FPS or 33.3 ms at 30 FPS.

Processing algorithm. In the first step of the algorithm each grayscale frame grabbed in real time from the video camera is smoothed with a Gaussian filter (fast computed using the CoreImage library). The output is then processed in one of two alternative operating modes: area-based or edge-based (Fig. 2).

In the area-based modality, the segmentation is performed considering the entire envelope (area) of the figure of the subject examined. In the edge-based modality, instead, an edge detection filter is applied to the image. The next step consists in a background subtraction technique computed to isolate the human figure from the ambient. In order to fulfill this task, each time the background changes, it has to be stored, area or edge based, with no human subject in front of the camera. If this

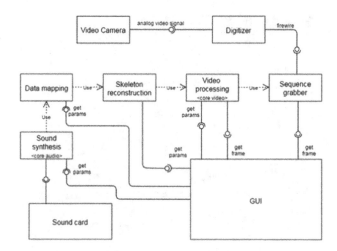

Fig. 1. System architecture.

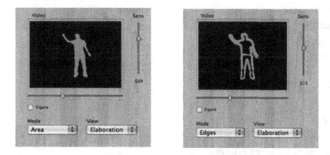

Fig. 2. Area-based (left) Edge-based (right)

background exists it is used in the following iterations of the algorithm and compared with the incoming frames containing the human figure using a dynamic threshold, obtaining a binary matrix. The average threshold used in this operation can be tuned by the operator in real time. It is not necessary to set again this sensitivity if the ambient light does not change. Finally, we apply an algorithm for removing unconnected small areas from the matrix, usually generated by image noise. The final binary image is then ready to be processed by the gesture tracking algorithm. The frame resolution is 320×240 pixels, full frame rate (e.g. 25 FPS) can be achieved because all the image filters are executed by the GPU. Starting from the binary raster matrix we apply an algorithm to detect a set of gesture parameters. This heuristic algorithm supposes that the segmented image obtained by the image elaboration process is a human figure, extracting data from it. This process starts searching a simplified model of the human figure, shown in the GUI (Fig. 3). Additional models for detailed parts of the body (face, hands) are currently under development, so that they can be used for more "zoomed" versions of the system. Starting from time dependent position of detected body joints we decided to compute the following parameters:

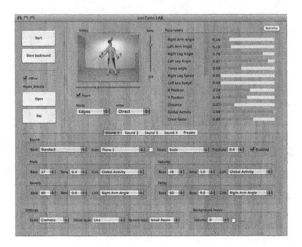

Fig. 3. Graphical User Interface

- *Right Arm angle*
- *Left Arm angle*
- *Right Leg angle*
- *Left Leg angle*
- *Torso angle*
- *Right Leg speed*
- *Left Leg speed*
- *Barycenter X*
- *Barycenter Y*
- *Distance of subject form camera.*

Their names are self-explaining. The distance from the camera actually is just an index related to the real distance: it is simply computed as a ratio between the frame height and the detected figure maximum height. The leg speed is computed analyzing the last couple of received frames; it is useful for triggering sounds with "kick-like" movements. We also compute these two additional parameters: global activity, crest factor.

The first is an indicator of overall quantity of movement (0.0 if the subject is standing still with no moments), while the second one is an indication of the concavity of the posture: (0.0 means that the subject is in standing position with arms kept along the body). Few optimizations are performed starting the frame analysis from an area centered in the last detected barycenter. Generally speaking, we tried to implement the detection algorithms in a very optimized way in order to maintain the target frame rate (25 FPS), minimizing the latency between gestures and sounds.

Sound Generation. The sound generation is based on the Mac OS CoreAudio library. We used the Audio Unit API for building a so called Audio graph. Four instances of DownLoadable Synthesizer (DLS) are mixed together in the final musical signal. These synthesizers produce sounds according to standard MIDI messages received from their virtual input ports. We added two digital effects (echo and Reverberation) to the final mix: for each synthesizer we can control the portion of its signal to be sent to these effects.

Each synthesizer module can load a bank of sounds (in the DLS or SF2 standard format) from the set installed in the system. The user can add his own sound banks, including the sounds he created, to the system. It is also possible to specify a background audio file, to be played together with the controlled sounds.

The mapper module translates the detected features into MIDI commands for the musical synthesizers. Each synthesizer works in independent way, and for each of them it is possible to select the instrument from different banks.

Each parameter of the sounds (pitch, volume, etc.) can be easily linked to the detected gesture parameters using the GUI. For example, we can link the Global Activity to the pitch: the faster you move the higher pitched notes you play. The synthesized MIDI notes are chosen from a user selectable scale: there's a large variety of them, ranging from the simplest ones (e.g. major and minor) to the more exotic ones. As an alternative, it is possible to select continuous pitch, instead of discrete notes: in this way the linked detected features controls the pitch in a "glissando" way. Sound can be triggered in a "Drum mode" way, too: the MIDI note C played when the linked parameters reach a selected threshold. All these links settings can be stored in presets, easily selectable from the operators.

3.2 Kinect Based Version

The experimentation has proven the positive effects so, in order to maintain its benefits, we developed a more user-friendly version to be used at home, avoiding the need of specialized personnel.

The user interface of this home version is greatly simplified compared to the video camera one and simply presents a series of easily selectable, not editable, presets. The body detection algorithm benefits from the use of Microsoft Kinect v2 SDK, which not requires the critical camera settings of the first version.

Microsoft Kinect. The Microsoft Kinect is a line of well-known motion sensing input devices originally created for Xbox 360 and Xbox One video game consoles and then Windows PCs. This device enables users to control and interact with their console/computer without the need for a game controller, through a natural user interface using gestures. The first Kinect version was using a structured infrared light approach while V2 (the version we used) is based on the Time-of-Flight (ToF) principle. Using these technologies, the device can compute a depth map of the environment. The Microsoft Kinect SDK libraries can process this depth map and extract the tridimensional coordinates of (up to) 26 joints of the human skeleton. Up to 6 skeletons can be tracked in real time. While Kinect V1 (which was considered during the development of the camera version) still suffered from large latency, the V2 partially solved this issue so that we finally decided to use it in the home version.

Software. This architecture of the SW, compared to the one described in Sect. 3.1, has the three modules Sequence Grabber Video Processor and Skeleton Reconstruction, replaced by routines developed with the Kinect SDK. Since this SDK provides only the spatial coordinates of the joints, we included a module for performing geometrical transformations on them, computing a set of features, basically the angles between body parts, that are invariant in relation to the body position and rotation. These features are then aggregated and mapped to sound with the same algorithm used in the camera based version.

Instead of supplying a rather complex GUI in which the user can create and customize presets (each one describing the relationship between motion and sounds) in this home version we include a set of predefined presets, easily accessible from a drop-down list. With this set we tried to cover a broad range of interaction modalities/gestures (arm motion, kicks, jumps etc.).

We included two special modes, designed for improving motor coordination. In the first one different movements trigger playbacks of a sampled voice pronouncing numbers: the subject has to sequence movements according to numbers order (randomly shuffled at each program launch). The second one is similar but we use fragments of sentences instead of numbers: here the user has to sequence these fragments to reconstruct a story (Fig. 4).

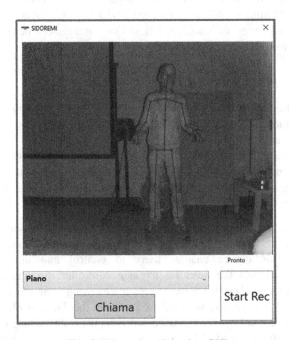

Fig. 4. Kinect based version GUI

This home version is intended to be used by the children's parents, not necessarily skilled. For this reason, they could eventually need a remote assistance. In order to provide a simple way to provide assistance we included a video chat mechanism in the software: the user, simply pressing a "call" button can make a video call to our technical staff.

Movement Recordings. We included a "record" button: pressing it all the child movements are recorded on disk for off-line analysis (for diagnostic purposes). The psychologist team that support the project suggested to analyze movements of the subject during the various sessions in order to objectively evaluate the effects of systems. We basically extract these features, as a function of time:

- Average of movements amount (whole body, upper, lower)
- Variance of movements amount (whole body, upper, lower)
- Average of movement speed (whole body, upper, lower)
- Variance of movements speed (whole body, upper, lower)
- Coordination (correlation between movements of different part of the body).

Since the concept of imitation is very important in the evaluation of autism spectrum disorder, we included an algorithm for computing *cross-correlation of movements* of two different bodies (the subject's one and the parent's one): this *similarity index* is strongly related to evidence of imitation (Fig. 5).

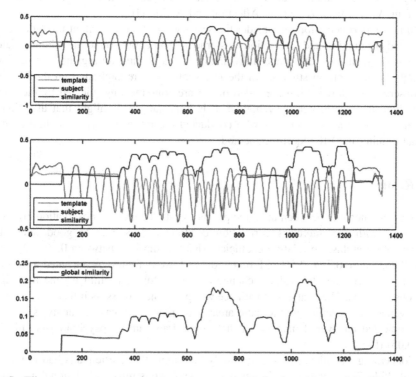

Fig. 5. Elbow movements in the two arms (upper graphs), for the subject and for his parent and (below) the resulting *similarity index*.

4 Experimentation

The experimentation [12] was performed in the school environment on 4 subjects (5–7 years, all males) diagnosed with Low-Functioning Autism (autism spectrum disorder, ASD). The weekly intervention lasted about 30 min. The children involved in the experimentation were evaluated in a cross sectional and follow up pilot study. Clinical features evaluated by mental health centers and information from the "Questionnaire on motor control and sensory elaboration" [13], compiled by parents, and from the "Short Sensory Profile" [14] filled up by the teachers were analyzed at baseline. Three clinical psychologists, not previously involved in the experimentation, analyzed the first eight videos of the intervention, completing an observation grid for every session (see Appendix A). The grid was structured ad hoc by the research team on the basis of the DIR Floortime model and technique in relation to the benchmarks of the main sensory profiles. This grid was partially taken from the questionnaire of Politi and colleagues [15] aimed at assessing the sensitivity of music in children affected by autism spectrum disorder. The instrument is made up of nineteen items relating to the child's behavior during the sessions and measured the characteristics of each sensory profile in terms of the "four A": Arousal, Attention, Affection and Action [16].

In this experimentation to consider the sensory profile of the infant that undergoes the sound stimulation and interaction was crucial. The choice of sound stimuli related to the movement has been made individually for each child during the first sessions through broad-spectrum stimuli. All the interventions were calibrated on the basis of the observations drawn from the video of the previous meeting, viewed by the reference clinician, a child neuropsychiatrist. It is important to highlight that the clinical reference as well as the operator who conducted the interventions with children had formal training in DIR Floortime method.

5 Results

The concordance rate between the three psychologists' behavioral observation grid was calculated with the interclass correlation coefficient. Moderate to good inter-rater agreement [interclass correlation coefficient (ICC) comprised between 0.596 (95% CI 0.41–0.853) and 0.799 (95% CI 0.489–0.933)] were found. A repeated measures design was performed to evaluate change over time for each child for the first eight sessions (T1–T8). The analysis of variance was performed to assess if there has been an improvement in specific symptomatic areas. The repeated measures analysis of variance indicated an overall increase of the scores drawn up by psychologists (T1–T8; $p < 0.05$) (Fig. 6).

Concerning statistical indexes our study highlights that participants had improved several skills. These variations in behavioral expressions reflect a relational evolution indicating the beginning of an opening attempt to someone no longer perceived as a threat but as someone from which to draw contentment, through playful interaction with the sounds. This pilot study demonstrates positive results: children developed skills in establishing joint attention, imitation of caregivers, communicating with gesture and symbols (Fig. 7).

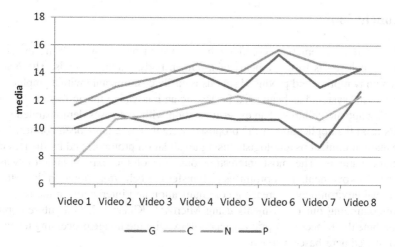

Fig. 6. Mean total scores of the behavior observation grid to assess change over time for each child (T1–T8).

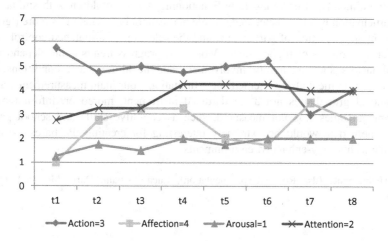

Fig. 7. Children's behavior (first eight videos) - Characteristics of each sensory profile in terms of Arousal, Attention, Affection and Action - From the observation grid of the first psychologist.

6   Conclusions

We described an interactive, computer based system based on real-time image processing, which reacts to movements of a human body playing sounds. The mapping between body motion and produced sounds is easily customizable with a graphical user interface. This system has been used for testing an innovative music-therapy technique for treating autistic children. The experimentation with real cases demonstrated several benefits from the application of the proposed system. These have been confirmed both by the team of clinical psychologists (using a validation protocol) and by the parents of the young patients. The most interesting outcome of the experimentation was the relational improvement. This promises to transfer the behavior shown in the setting to the external environment, increasing communication and interaction in the real world. We are continuing our experiments using Microsoft Kinect v.2. Our future approach will combine the Kinect's proprietary technology with the image processing techniques used in the camera based version.

The project addressed many challenges. Each autistic child is unique in the sense that improvements in abilities are very subjective and some study limitations have to be mentioned: first of all, the small size and the non-homogeneity of the sample; this is due to the difficulty of enrolling Low-Functioning Autism children with similar profiles. Participation is self-selected and sample bias cannot be excluded. A more rigorous assessment and selection of participants and the selection of a matched control group will guarantee results of higher value. Moreover, progress trends could depend upon external factors such as family involvement and health/treatment conditions. The outcome measurement also presented some limitations: our main measurement was the observational grid that is not a standardized instrument; moreover, information on important outcomes was not measured, such as cognitive skills and school performance. These data would be extremely interesting for creating the bases for using accessible technology-enhanced environments.

Acknowledgement. Elsa Rossi (Experimentation), Luca Bastiani, Dario Menicagli (Video analysis).

Appendix A: Observation Grid

Video Observation Grid

Section 1

Name and surname of the child:

Date of birth: _ _ / _ _ / _ _ _ _   Date of observation: _ _ / _ _ / _ _ _ _

Name and surname of the observer:

Time of permanence in the setting (in minutes):

Section 2			Sensory profile
The child listens and responds to different sounds	**Yes** (1)	**No** (0)	Arousal
The child appears absent	**Yes** (0)	**No** (1)	Attention
The child introduces original elements in the context	**Yes** (1)	**No** (0)	Action
The child is distracted	**Yes** (0)	**No** (1)	Attention
The child produces a variety of sounds	**Yes** (1)	**No** (0)	Action
Eye contact with the operator	**Yes** (1)	**No** (0)	Attention
The child carries out maneuvers of avoidance	**Yes** (0)	**No** (1)	Action
Physical contact with the operator	**Yes** (1)	**No** (0)	Affection
Aggressive physical modalities	**Yes** (0)	**No** (1)	Action
Affective / emotional physical modalities	**Yes** (1)	**No** (0)	Action
Rigid muscle tone	**Yes** (0)	**No** (1)	Action
Proper to the interaction muscle tone	**Yes** (1)	**No** (0)	Action
Verbal communicative effectiveness of distress signal behavior	**Yes** (1)	**No** (0)	Affection
Non verbal communicative effectiveness of distress signal behavior	**Yes** (1)	**No** (0)	Affection
Particular sensitivity to sound frequencies and / or to the nature of sounds	**Yes** (1)	**No** (0)	Arousal
Sonorous or motory imitative behaviors	**Yes** (1)	**No** (0)	Attention
Attention shared with the operator	**Yes** (1)	**No** (0)	Attention
Motor stereotypies	**Yes** (0)	**No** (1)	Action
Emotional attunement with the operator	**Yes** (1)	**No** (0)	Affection
Score (please, sum scores in the brackets)			

References

1. Magrini, M., Carboni, A., Salvetti, O., Curzio, O.: An auditory feedback based system for treating autism spectrum disorder. In: Proceedings of the 3rd 2015 Workshop on ICTs for Improving Patients Rehabilitation Research Techniques. REHAB 2015, pp. 30–33. ACM, New York (2015)
2. Mohamed, A.O., Courbulay, V.: Attention analysis in interactive software for children with autism. In: Proceedings of the 8th International ACM SIGACCESS Conference on Computers and Accessibility, Portland (2006)
3. Kozima, H., Nakagawa, C., Yasuda, Y.: Interactive robots for communication-care: a case-study in autism therapy. In: International IEEE Workshop on Robot and Human Interactive Communication (2005)

4. Villafuerte, L., Markova, M., Jorda, S.: Acquisition of social abilities through musical tangible user interface: children with autism spectrum condition and the reactable. In: Proceedings of CHI 2012 Extended Abstracts on Human Factors in Computing Systems. CHI EA 2012, pp. 745–760. ACM, New York (2012)
5. Riva, D., Bulgheroni, S., Zappella, M.: Neurobiology, Diagnosis & Treatment in Autism: An Update. John Libbey Eurotex (2013)
6. Pajareya, K., Nopmaneejumruslers, K.: A pilot randomized con-trolled trial of DIR/Floortime™ parent training intervention for pre-school children with autistic spectrum disorders. Autism **15**(5), 563–577 (2011)
7. Solomon, R., et al.: Pilot study of a parent training program for young children with autism the PLAY Project Home Consultation program. Autism **11**(3), 205–224 (2007)
8. Wing, L., Gould, J.: Severe impairments of social interaction and associated abnormalities in children: epidemiology and classification. J. Autism Dev. Disord. **9**, 11–29 (1979)
9. Vismara, V.A., Rogers, S.J.: Behavioral treatments in autism spectrum disorder: what do we know? Annu. Rev. Clin. Psychol. **6**, 447–468 (2010)
10. Kanner, L.: Autistic disturbances of affective contact. Nerv. Child **2**, 217–250 (1943)
11. Greenspan, S., Wieder, S.: The Child with Special Needs. Perseus Publishing, New York (1998)
12. Magrini, M., et.al.: Progetto "SI RE MI" Sistema di Rieducazione Espressiva del Movimento e dell'Interazione.. Autismo e disturbi dello sviluppo, Erickson (2015)
13. DeGangi, G., Berck, R.: DeGangi-Berck: Test of Sensory Integration. Western Psychological Services, Los Angeles (1983)
14. Dunn, W.: Sensory Profile-School Companion. Psychological Corporation, San Antonio (2006)
15. Politi, P., Emanuele, E., e Grassi, M.: The invisible orchestra project. development of the "Playing-in-Touch" (PiT) questionnaire. Neuroendocrinol. Lett. **33**(5), 552–558 (2012)
16. Meini, C., Guiot, G., Sindelar, M.T.: Autismo e musica. Il modello Floortime nei disturbi della comunicazione e della relazione, Erickson (2012)

Using Wii Balance Board to Evaluate Software Based on Kinect2

Zhihan Lv$^{(\boxtimes)}$, Vicente Penades, Sonia Blasco, Javier Chirivella,
and Pablo Gagliardo

FIVAN, Valencia, Spain
lvzhihan@gmail.com

Abstract. A balance measurement software based on Kinect2 sensor is evaluated by comparing to Wii balance board in numerical analysis level, and further improved according to the consideration of BFP (Body fat percentage) values of the user. Several person with different body types are involved into the test. The algorithm is improved by comparing the body type of the user to the 'golden-standard' body type. The evaluation results of the optimized algorithm preliminarily prove the reliability of the software.

Keywords: Virtual reality · Center of mass · Balance · Kinect · WBB

1 Introduction

The center of pressure (CoP) is also known as center of mass (CoM). It is measured by different methods according to different technical levels in different age. The methods which are already applied in clinic include Balance Error Scoring System (BESS), 'gold-standard' laboratory-grade force plate (FP), wii lance board (WBB). Our research is to measure to what extend the kinect balance measurement (KBM) method can be accepted by clinical utilization. In kinesiology research community, currently, there are several kinds of measurements methods for comparison the 'gold-standard' laboratory-grade force plate (FP) to wii balance board (WBB) presented. There are some measurement results recorded in current literature. [53] compared the game scores provided by Wii to traditional balance measures. [7] wanted to see if traditional balance measures (like Center of Pressure velocity) were reliable on the wii balance board and valid compared to a forceplate, so they bypassed the games and simply collected the raw data. [1] performed a standard measurement uncertainty analysis to provide the repeatability and accuracy of the WBB force and CoP measurements. In summary, the data from a wii balance board is valid and reliable [4,7,16] but the game scores that are produced are not [53]. Moreover, WBB may be useful for low-resolution measurements, but should not be considered as a replacement for laboratory-grade force plates. Therefore, WBB is enough accurate to measure

© Springer International Publishing AG 2017
H.M. Fardoun et al. (Eds.): REHAB 2015, CCIS 665, pp. 59–68, 2017.
https://doi.org/10.1007/978-3-319-69694-2_6

our athome rehabilitation application using kinect, but the customized software is expected to be developed.

In robotics research community, a series of researches have been already done about comparison kinect balance measurement (KBM) and Vicon balance measurement (VBM) to wii balance board (WBB) [17–19].

The Wii Balance Board is shaped like a household body scale, with a plain white top and light gray bottom. It runs on four AA batteries as a power source, which can power the board for about 60 h. The board uses Bluetooth technology and contains four pressure sensors that are used to measure the user's center of balance–the location of the intersection between an imaginary line drawn vertically through the center of mass and the surface of the Balance Board–and weight. In an interview conducted by gaming web site IGN, Shigeru Miyamoto stated that the Balance Board's ability to measure weight is probably more accurate than that of a typical bathroom scale. The WBB consists of a rigid platform with four uni-axial vertical force transducers located in the feet at the corners of the board, one transducer per foot. Each transducer is a load cell consisting of a cantilevered metal bar with a strain gauge that converts applied force into a voltage that is digitized and transmitted wirelessly by electronics in the WBB. The WBB has been demonstrated to be a reliable and valid instrument for the assessment of other physical characteristics such as balance and reaction-time. In 2014, an American research group demonstrated that both new and used WBB recorded static forces accurately in a laboratory setting. Inspired by these findings, researchers at Aalborg University Hospital have developed software that enabled isometric strength recordings to be performed using the WBB. This software has shown high reproducibility and concurrent validity for measuring isometric muscle strength in the lower limbs.

In the experiment, the WBB was placed on top of the FP to obtain measurement from both devices at the same time, which is set as the same as the method1 proposed in kinesiology research community. The person were instructed to stand on top of the FP and WBB and hold 40 static postures, each lasting 5s. [19] mentioned that the reason to measure the KBM is that the improper lighting, loose fitting clothes, and large objects which surround the subject can adversely influence the skeleton fitting. In our kinect2 based KBM method, we find age, height, body type of the person as well as the error in foot tip position measurement also affect the CoP measurement results slightly. This paper is the extended version of our work on Rehab2015 [40].

The purpose of our measurement is different from the previous measurements, since they just compared 'gold-standard' laboratory-grade force plate (FP) to a game controller wii balance board (WBB). It is undeniable that they proved that WBB can replace Balance Error Scoring System (BESS) which is used for assessing the balance as subjective method for past years. Even some productions are developed based their research, such as BtrackS [15] which is proved to reach the same level as WBB. But our KBM method is based on totally different measurement algorithm theory, implementation technology and suitable device context. We are using the range image data captured by kinect2 device in real-time, and further measure the CoP by our customized algorithm based on optical theory. The Wii balance board can cannot measure any information about the weight and CoP onside the device, while the kinect can get full information appeared in the camera view, but is not enable to retrieve the weight information since it is a non-contact sensor. Nonetheless, the same characteristics of both devices are that they have specialty or potential to measure CoP, but cannot measure density information by any direct or indirect methods. Therefore, the robotics research community attracts our attention. The 'Center of mass calculation by kinect' [18] uses SESC as the core algorithm to solve the calculation of CoM. This work has been compared to some other work: 1. FP; 2. WBB; 3. Kinect; 4. Vicon (High quality camera); 5. Winter's method.

2   System

In our research, we will consider the previous proposed methods and results in both kinesiology research community and robotics research community, and design our particular measurement method according to our algorithm theory, device condition and clinical needs. The hardware devices we currently owned include: 1. WBB; 2. Several Kinect2. The algorithm that is similar with our algorithm is mentioned in literature [21,26], which is so-called segmentation methods, also known as kinematic methods. The problem that 'performed mainly on cadavers or in live, young and fit individuals' is also mentioned [13,54]. Some solutions are also discussed [45], which is 'should be adjusted for age, sex and fitness level'.

3   Evaluation and Improving

The evaluation is conducted along with the improving process. The evaluation process includes several stages. During the evaluation, the subject should place the stance limb in the center of the Wii balance board and place his or her hands on the hips and eyes open. Next, he or she will reach as far as possible in the 3 reach directions with the contralateral limb. Reach distance was defined as the farthest point that an individual could touch without accepting weight and while maintaining balance through the return to a bilateral stance.

Four person with different body type were involved into the test. The purpose of this session is to find the relation between the body type with the errors of CoM calculation. Body segment inertial parameters (BSIPs) are important data in biomechanics. BSIPs have been measured by different methods, e.g. [3,52] employs a whole body dual energy X-ray absorptiometry scan, [5] employs a motion capture system and two forceplates, [8,9] employs a single kinect, [12] employs several digital cameras, [20] proposed a validation method to evaluate BSIPs.

Our balance measurement algorithm is using segmentation method, based on which, the weight of each segment's CoM position is the ratio of the segments to total body mass. BSIPs are the parameters for this purpose. It's already proved that BSIPs are depending on the age, gender and body type and some researches have modified the classic BSIPs based on this theory [2,13,14,45,47,58] even concerning the effects of weight loss in obese individuals [43] and individuals of different morphology [10], as well as composite concerning. Methods relying on imagery have the drawback that the segmentation of body parts is complex, thus affecting significantly the BSIP values [20]. Indeed, the BSIP depend on the relative amount of bone, muscle and adipose tissue in a body segment which underlie structural and temporalchanges when aging or caused by pathology or training [25,48]. [24,44,46] have measured the extent to which errors in predicting body segment parameters could influence biomechanical analysis of human motion, predicted joint moment and joint kinetics.

This research is used to explorer the relationship between some metrics with the BSIPs and further improve the calculation of CoM. The most important factor is Body type, which is also known as body shape. Body shape is affected by body fat distribution, which is correlated to current levels of sex hormones. There are some existing metrics to evaluate the body type, such as BMI (Body Mass Index), BFP (Body fat percentage), BVI (Body Volume Index), WHR (Waist-hip ratio), WhtR (waist-to-height ratio). The series of images of the results indicate that the normalized distances on X-axis between the CoM of Kinect and WBB haven't obvious regular patterns. While the normalized distances on Y-axis between the CoM of Kinect and WBB have the similar orbit that the normalized CoM of WBB is always after the normalized CoM of Kinect. It also reveals that the normalized distances on Y-axis between the CoM of Kinect and WBB depend on BFP. Because the order of the distances for the three subjects are $B(m = 67, sd = 11) > C(m = 48, sd = 18) > A(m = 13, sd = 11)$, which is the same as the order of $BFP(B(30.96) > C(23.39) > A(19.51))$. The order of other metrics (i.e. BMI, WHR, WhtR) have different order.

BFP is also written as $BF\%$, which is usually measured by physical device, such as underwater weighing, whole-body air displacement plethysmography, near-infrared interactance, dual energy X-ray absorptiometry. In our application scene, the physical device is not suitable. So we employes the formula derived from previous researches' statistic results [50].

According to this supposed regular pattern, we proposed a new improvement plan, which considers the relative value of BFP of the player comparing to BFP of golden standard player (A). We will start from the derivation of a linear relation between BFP and the distance on Y-axis to represent the regular pattern. In contrast to the previous test for individual subject, we have considered the body types of three health people with different ages, height, weight this time. According to the BFP as well as the regular pattern indicated in the test results, the new refined formula for reducing error of distance between CoM of Kinect and WBB is proposed.

The evaluation of the new formula is conducted. Since the body type of A is supposed as golden standard in our research, so the error of distance remains the value (m = 13, sd = 11) after being refined by the new formula. This distance for B is vastly changed from (m = 67, sd = 11) to (m = 10, sd = 8). The result for

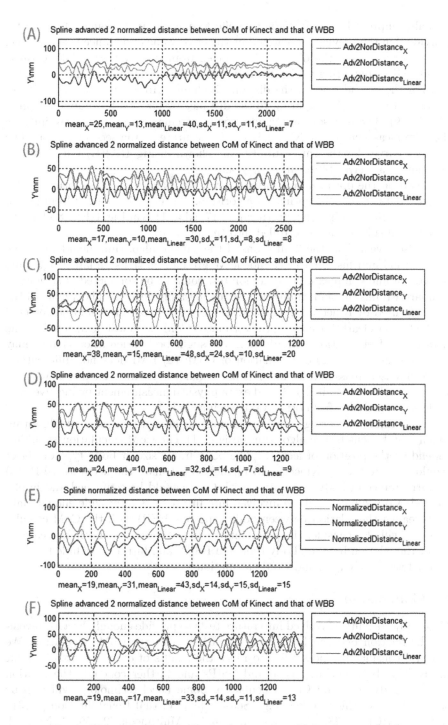

Fig. 1. The evaluation results for four person. (Color figure online)

C is also improved, even if it's not so effective as the improvement formula for individual in the previous research, but the error value of distance is acceptable. For the first session, the distance is changed from (m = 32, sd = 20) to (m = 15, sd = 10), comparing to the distance by formula for individual (m = 13, sd = 10). For the second session, the distance is changed from (m = 48, sd = 18) to (mean = 10, sd = 7) comparing to the distance by formula for individual (m = 12, sd = 9). The first session includes some extreme actions, so we can imagine that the measurement by Kinect is not so accurate as the second session. The distance curves for the three subjects are shown in Fig. 1(A)(B)(C)(D), where blue curves are error of distance on Y-axis.

Based on the optimization formula proposed before, we use another health people's data to test the optimized algorithm. The error is changed from (mean = 31, sd = 15) (in Fig. 1(E)) to (mean = 17, sd = 11) (in Fig. 1(F)). So far, the errors of all subjects are controlled into (mean = 20).

It also reveal that, the limitations of the current algorithm include: (1) The player stand and his/her feet cannot leave ground. So the standard single limb stance test and complex random-action test couldn't be conducted. The golden-standard FP has the same limitation, so it's not a big deal; (2) The quality of the data captured by Kinect is significant. The feet of the player should be detected by the Kinect clearly, otherwise, the estimated CoM value will be affected by the error of the feet positions. In addition, the slight body orientation change may lead to incorrect results of estimation of CoM; (3) BMI does not differentiate between muscle mass and fat mass, is particularly inaccurate for people who are very fit or athletic. While BFP need extra physical measurement by inconvenient devices or concluded from other value such as WHR;

Furthermore, we bring some suggestions to improve the current algorithm which may benefit future algorithm design: (1) The CoM calculation shouldn't depend on the position of feet; (2) The body frame size or body type of player should be detected by Kinect, and further to calculate the accurate BFP; (3) The irrelevance of body orientation with CoM should be confirmed and implemented. More subjects will be involved into future tests to provide enough data for revealing the relation between body type (i.e. BFP) with the CoM calculation. We will also consider the possibility to reuse the results of other researches about the relation between body type and BSIPs and further conclude the relation between body type and CoM calculation.

4   Conclusion

More subjects will be involved into future tests to provide enough data for revealing the relation between body type (i.e. BFP) with the CoM calculation. We will also consider the possibility to reuse the results of other researches about the relation between body type and BSIPs and further conclude the relation between body type and CoM calculation. Some novel technology will also be used to improve this research, e.g., Sensors [55], Virtual Rehabilitation [29, 31–33, 39, 41], HCI [34–38, 49], Video Game [6, 42], Multimedia [28, 56, 57] Network and Distributed Computing [22, 23, 27, 30, 51], Optimization Algorithm [11].

Acknowledgment. The authors thank to LanPercept, a Marie Curie Initial Training Network funded through the 7th EU Framework Programme (316748).

References

1. Bartlett, H.L., Ting, L.H., Bingham, J.T.: Accuracy of force and center of pressure measures of the Wii Balance Board. Gait Posture **39**(1), 224–228 (2014)
2. Challis, J.H., Winter, S.L., Kuperavage, A.J.: Comparison of male and female lower limb segment inertial properties. J. Biomech. **45**(15), 2690–2692 (2012)
3. Chambers, A.J., Sukits, A.L., McCrory, J.L., Cham, R.: The effect of obesity and gender on body segment parameters in older adults. Clin. Biomech. **25**(2), 131–136 (2010)
4. Chang, J.O., Levy, S.S., Seay, S.W., Goble, D.J.: An alternative to the balance error scoring system: using a low-cost balance board to improve the validity/reliability of sports-related concussion balance testing. Clin. J. Sport Med. **24**(3), 256–262 (2014)
5. Chen, S.-C., Hsieh, H.-J., Lu, T.-W., Tseng, C.-H.: A method for estimating subject-specific body segment inertial parameters in human movement analysis. Gait Posture **33**(4), 695–700 (2011)
6. Chen, Z., Huang, W., Lv, Z.: Towards a face recognition method based on uncorrelated discriminant sparse preserving projection. Multimedia Tools Appl., 1–15 (2015)
7. Clark, R.A., Bryant, A.L., Pua, Y., McCrory, P., Bennell, K., Hunt, M.: Validity and reliability of the nintendo wii balance board for assessment of standing balance. Gait Posture **31**(3), 307–310 (2010)
8. Clarkson, S., Choppin, S., Hart, J., Heller, B., Wheat, J.: Calculating body segment inertia parameters from a single rapid scan using the Microsoft Kinect. In: Proceedings of the 3rd International Conference on 3D Body Scanning Technologies, pp. 153–163 (2012)
9. Clarkson, S., Wheat, J., Heller, B., Choppin, S.: Assessing the suitability of the Microsoft Kinect for calculating person specific body segment parameters. In: Agapito, L., Bronstein, M.M., Rother, C. (eds.) ECCV 2014. LNCS, vol. 8925, pp. 372–385. Springer, Cham (2015). doi:10.1007/978-3-319-16178-5_26
10. Damavandi, M., Farahpour, N., Allard, P.: Determination of body segment masses and centers of mass using a force plate method in individuals of different morphology. Med. Eng. Phys. **31**(9), 1187–1194 (2009)
11. Dang, S., Ju, J., Matthews, D., Feng, X., Zuo, C.: Efficient solar power heating system based on lenticular condensation. In: 2014 International Conference on Information Science, Electronics and Electrical Engineering (ISEEE), vol. 2, pp. 736–739, April 2014
12. Davidson, P.L., Wilson, S.J., Wilson, B.D., Chalmers, D.J.: Estimating subject-specific body segment parameters using a 3-Dimensional modeller program. J. Biomech. **41**(16), 3506–3510 (2008)
13. De Leva, P.: Adjustments to zatsiorsky-seluyanov's segment inertia parameters. J. Biomech. **29**(9), 1223–1230 (1996)
14. Dumas, R., Cheze, L., Verriest, J.-P.: Adjustments to Mcconville et al. and Young et al. body segment inertial parameters. J. Biomech. **40**(3), 543–553 (2007)
15. Goble, D.: Btracks (2015). http://balancetrackingsystems.com

16. Goble, D.J., Cone, B.L., Fling, B.W.: Using the wii fit as a tool for balance assessment and neurorehabilitation: the first half decade of Wii-search. J. Neuroeng. Rehabil. **11**(12), 0003–11 (2014)
17. Gonzalez, A., Fraisse, P., Hayashibe, M.: Adaptive interface for personalized center of mass self-identification in home rehabilitation. IEEE Sensors J. **15**(5), 2814–2823 (2015)
18. González, A., Hayashibe, M., Bonnet, V., Fraisse, P.: Whole body center of mass estimation with portable sensors: Using the statically equivalent serial chain and a kinect. Sensors **14**(9), 16955–16971 (2014)
19. González, A., Hayashibe, M., Fraisse, P.: Estimation of the center of mass with Kinect and Wii Balance Board. In: 2012 IEEE/RSJ International Conference on Intelligent Robots and Systems (IROS), pp. 1023–1028. IEEE (2012)
20. Hansen, C., Venture, G., Rezzoug, N., Gorce, P., Isableu, B.: An individual and dynamic body segment inertial parameter validation method using ground reaction forces. J. Biomech. **47**(7), 1577–1581 (2014)
21. Jaffrey, M.A.: Estimating centre of mass trajectory and subject-specific body segment parameters using optimisation approaches. PhD thesis, Victoria University (2008)
22. Jiang, D., Xu, Z., Lv, Z.: A multicast delivery approach with minimum energy consumption for wireless multi-hop networks. Telecommun. Syst., 1–12 (2015)
23. Jiang, D., Ying, X., Han, Y., Lv, Z.: Collaborative multi-hop routing in cognitive wireless networks.Wireless Pers. Commun., 1–23 (2015)
24. Kiernan, D., Walsh, M., O'Sullivan, R., O'Brien, T., Simms, C.: The influence of estimated body segment parameters on predicted joint kinetics during diplegic cerebral palsy gait. J. Biomech. **47**(1), 284–288 (2014)
25. Kyle, U.G., Genton, L., Hans, D., Karsegard, V.L., Michel, J.-P., Slosman, D.O., Pichard, C.: Total body mass, fat mass, fat-free mass, and skeletal muscle in older people: cross-sectional differences in 60-year-old persons. J. Am. Geriatr. Soc. **49**(12), 1633–1640 (2001)
26. Lafond, D., Duarte, M., Prince, F.: Comparison of three methods to estimate the center of mass during balance assessment. J. Biomech. **37**(9), 1421–1426 (2004)
27. Li, T., Zhou, X., Brandstatter, K., Zhao, D., Wang, K., Rajendran, A., Zhang, Z., Raicu, I.: ZHT: a light-weight reliable persistent dynamic scalable zero-hop distributed hash table. In: 2013 IEEE 27th International Symposium on Parallel & Distributed Processing (IPDPS), pp. 775–787. IEEE (2013)
28. Liu, Y., Yang, J., Meng, Q., Lv, Z., Song, Z., Gao, Z.: Stereoscopic image quality assessment method based on binocular combination saliency model. Sig. Process. **125**, 237–248 (2016)
29. Lv, Z.: Bringing immersive enjoyment to hyperbaric oxygen chamber users using virtual reality glasses. In: Proceedings of the 3rd 2015 Workshop on ICTs for Improving Patients Rehabilitation Research Techniques, pp. 156–159. ACM (2015)
30. Lv, Z., Chirivella, J., Gagliardo, P.: Bigdata oriented multimedia mobile health applications. J. Med. Syst. **40**(5), 1–10 (2016)
31. Lv, Z., Esteve, C., Chirivella, J., Gagliardo, P.: Clinical feedback and technology selection of game based dysphonic rehabilitation tool. In 9th International Conference on Pervasive Computing Technologies for Healthcare (PervasiveHealth2015). IEEE (2015)
32. Lv, Z., Esteve, C., Chirivella, J., Gagliardo, P.: A game based assistive tool for rehabilitation of dysphonic patients. In: 2015 3rd IEEE VR International Workshop on Virtual and Augmented Assistive Technology (VAAT), pp. 9–14, March 2015

33. Lv, Z., Esteve, C., Chirivella, J., Gagliardo, P.: Serious game based dysphonic reha-
    bilitation tool. In: International Conference on Virtual Rehabilitation (ICVR2015).
    IEEE (2015)
34. Lv, Z., Feng, L., Li, H., Feng, S.: Hand-free motion interaction on Google glass.
    In: SIGGRAPH Asia 2014 Mobile Graphics and Interactive Applications. ACM
    (2014)
35. Lv, Z., Feng, S., Feng, L., Li, H.: Extending touch-less interaction on vision based
    wearable device. In: 2015 IEEE Virtual Reality (VR), pp. 231–232, March 2015
36. Lv, Z., Feng, S., Khan, M.S.L., Ur Réhman, S., Li, H.: Foot motion sensing: aug-
    mented game interface based on foot interaction for smartphone. In: CHI 2014
    Extended Abstracts on Human Factors in Computing Systems, pp. 293–296. ACM
    (2014)
37. Lv, Z., Halawani, A., Feng, S., Ur Réhman, S.: Multimodal hand and foot ges-
    ture interaction for handheld devices. ACM Trans. Multimedia Comput. Commun.
    Appl. (TOMM) **11**(1s), 1–19 (2014)
38. Lv, Z., Halawani, A., Feng, S., Ur Réhman, S., Li, H.: Touch-less interactive aug-
    mented reality game on vision-based wearable device. Pers. Ubiquit. Comput.
    19(3–4), 551–567 (2015)
39. Lv, Z., Li, H.: Imagining in-air interaction for Hemiplegia sufferer. In: International
    Conference on Virtual Rehabilitation (ICVR2015). IEEE (2015)
40. Lv, Z., Penades, V., Blasco, S., Chirivella, J., Gagliardo, P.: Comparing Kinect2
    based balance measurement software to Wii Balance Board. In: Proceedings of
    the 3rd 2015 Workshop on ICTs for improving Patients Rehabilitation Research
    Techniques, pp. 50–53. ACM (2015)
41. Lv, Z., Penades, V., Blasco, S., Chirivella, J., Gagliardo, P.: Intuitive evaluation
    of Kinect2 based balance measurement software. In: Proceedings of the 3rd 2015
    Workshop on ICTs for improving Patients Rehabilitation Research Techniques, pp.
    62–65. ACM (2015)
42. Lv, Z., Tek, A., Da Silva, F., Empereur-Mot, C., Chavent, M., Baaden, M.: Game
    on, science-how video game technology may help biologists tackle visualization
    challenges. PLoS One **8**(3), 57990 (2013)
43. Matrangola, S.L., Madigan, M.L., Nussbaum, M.A., Ross, R., Davy, K.P.: Changes
    in body segment inertial parameters of obese individuals with weight loss. J. Bio-
    mech. **41**(15), 3278–3281 (2008)
44. Nguyen, T.C., Reynolds, K.J.: The effect of variability in body segment parameters
    on joint moment using Monte Carlo Simulations. Gait Posture **39**(1), 346–353
    (2014)
45. Pavol, M.J., Owings, T.M., Grabiner, M.D.: Body segment inertial parameter esti-
    mation for the general population of older adults. J. Biomech. **35**(5), 707–712
    (2002)
46. Pearsall, D., Costigan, P.: The effect of segment parameter error on gait analysis
    results. Gait Posture **9**(3), 173–183 (1999)
47. Pryce, R., Kriellaars, D.: Body segment inertial parameters and low back load in
    individuals with central adiposity. J. Biomech. **47**(12), 3080–3086 (2014)
48. Rao, G., Amarantini, D., Berton, E., Favier, D.: Influence of body segments' para-
    meters estimation models on inverse dynamics solutions during gait. J. Biomech.
    39(8), 1531–1536 (2006)
49. Khan, M.S.L., Lu, Z., Li, H., et al.: Head orientation modeling: geometric head
    pose estimation using monocular camera. In: The 1st IEEE/IIAE International
    Conference on Intelligent Systems and Image Processing 2013, pp. 149–153 (2013)

50. Trefethen, N.: New BMI (body mass index) (2013). https://people.maths.ox.ac. uk/trefethen/bmi.html
51. Wang, K., Zhou, X., Chen, H., Lang, M., Raicu, I.: Next generation job management systems for extreme-scale ensemble computing. In: Proceedings of the 23rd International Symposium on High-Performance Parallel and Distributed Computing, pp. 111–114. ACM (2014)
52. Wicke, J., Dumas, G.A., Costigan, P.A.: A comparison between a new model and current models for estimating trunk segment inertial parameters. J. Biomech. **42**(1), 55–60 (2009)
53. Wikstrom, E.A.: Validity and reliability of nintendo Wii Fit Balance Scores. J. Athletic Training **47**(3), 306 (2012)
54. Winter, D.A.: Biomechanics and Motor Control of Human Movement. Wiley, New York (2009)
55. Yang, J., Chen, B., Zhou, J., Lv, Z.: A low-power and portable biomedical device for respiratory monitoring with a stable power source. Sensors **15**(8), 19618–19632 (2015)
56. Yang, J., Lin, Y., Gao, Z., Lv, Z., Wei, W., Song, H.: Quality index for stereoscopic images by separately evaluating adding and subtracting. PLoS One **10**(12), e0145800 (2015)
57. Yu, J., Skaff, S., Peng, L., Imai, F.: Leveraging knowledge-based inference for material classification. In: Proceedings of the 23rd Annual ACM Conference on Multimedia Conference, pp. 1243–1246. ACM (2015)
58. Zatsiorsky, V., Seluyanov, V., Chugunova, L.: Methods of determining mass-inertial characteristics of human body segments. Contemp. Problems Biomech. **272**, 291 (1990)

Cognitive Improvement via mHealth for Patients Recovering from Substance Use Disorder

B. Rosa[1,2], J. Oliveira[1,2(✉)], P. Gamito[1,2], P. Lopes[1,2], D. Morais[1,2], R. Brito[1,2], C. Caçoête[3], A. Leandro[3], T. Almeida[3], and H. Oliveira[3]

[1] EPCV/Lusophone University, Campo Grande, 376, Lisbon, Portugal
{beatriz.rosa,jorge.oliveira,pedro.gamito,paulo.jorge,
diogo.morais,rodrigo.brito}@ulusofona.pt
[2] COPELABS/Lusophone University, Campo Grande, 376, Lisbon, Portugal
[3] Ares do Pinhal Addiction Rehabilitation Association, Rua Gil Vicente, 62A, Lisbon, Portugal
{cristiana.cacoete,andre.leandro,teresa.almeida,
hugo.oliveira}@aresdopinhal.pt

Abstract. Heroin addiction has a negative impact on cognitive functions, which may also contribute to poorer treatment outcomes in drug addition. Traditional cognitive rehabilitation approaches suffer from limited motivational appeal and are relatively cumbersome to carry out. Thus, we report a study testing the efficacy of an alternative mHealth approach using tablets and serious games to stimulate cognitive functions in recovering addicts. This approach was tested in a sample 14 male heroin addicts undergoing a rehabilitation program for heroin addiction as inpatients at a local NGO. The exercises for cognitive training were based on serious games running on tablets. The results showed improvements in cognitive functioning between baseline and follow-up assessments in frontal lobe functions, verbal memory and sustained attention, as well as in some aspects of cognitive flexibility, decision-making and depression. Patients in cognitive training had a higher proportion of positive outcomes related to indicators of verbal memory cognitive flexibility than patients not in training. Overall results are promising but still require randomized control trials to determine the efficiency of this approach as an alternative to cognitive rehabilitation programs in heroin addicts.

Keywords: Cognitive training · mHealth · Heroin addiction

1 Introduction

Cognitive training and rehabilitation programmes are used to improve cognitive recovery from impairments following brain trauma, strokes, and addiction. They are fundamental in helping individuals recover their ability to function normally in their daily lives. Traditional cognitive rehabilitation and training techniques, however, are expensive and cumbersome, and not widely accessible. Emerging ICT-based techniques have been taking advantage of the widespread availability and motivational appeal of digital technology to broaden the access and efficiency of cognitive training. However, these techniques need to be tested in a broad variety of clinical populations with cognitive impairments in order to

© Springer International Publishing AG 2017
H.M. Fardoun et al. (Eds.): REHAB 2015, CCIS 665, pp. 69–82, 2017.
https://doi.org/10.1007/978-3-319-69694-2_7

assess their efficacy and efficiency. Here we report a pilot study on the use of an ICT-based cognitive training programme for the cognitive rehabilitation of recovering heroin addicts.

1.1 Heroin Addiction and Cognitive Impairment

Addiction to heroin is a worldwide problem. Opioid overdose is estimated to cause 69.000 deaths each year [1], and heroin use in the United States has been increasing in the past years, from 214,000 in 2002 to 467,000 in 2012 [2]. Heroin use also has well-documented negative effects on cognitive functions: morphine diacetate (the heroin molecule, which is a synthesis of a morphine molecule with two acetyl groups), when injected, has the ability to easily cross the blood-brain barrier due to the presence of the acetyl groups [3]; once in the brain, it loses the two acetyl groups, turning into morphine, which induces relaxation and intense euphoria [4]. The regular use of heroin stimulates the production of such receptors, leading to greater tolerance and dependence; increased doses are required to achieve the initial levels of relaxation and euphoria [5]. This modification on the receptors, and on the circuits that mediate the interaction of the morphine molecule, alters the activity of the limbic system, interfering with emotional and cognitive processing [6]. Data from previous studies [7] suggested that long-term heroin users had significantly lower telomerase activity, which is an important index of cellular aging probably indicating that heroin abuse accelerates the biological aging. This may also suggest that low level of telomerase is associated with compromised structural integrity of the right dorsolateral prefrontal cortex. In line with these suggestions, neuroimaging studies also reported a pattern of prefrontal dysfunction in addict abusers [8] and reduced activation of the dorsal anterior cingulate cortex [6]. As the prefrontal regions play a critical role in the organization of cognitive and behavioural processes as well as in the adaptation of environment [9, 10], findings from biological and neurological studies provide information that contributes for an accurate understanding of cognitive and emotional processes of heroin-dependent subjects.

Studies have consistently shown that heroin consumption impacts on several domains of cognition. Some authors [11–13] stressed that in opioid users, deficits are observed in attention, concentration, recall, and visuospatial skills, however, in at long-term, deficits will be reflected on executive dysfunctions as well [13]. Because executive functions refers a set of cognitive dimensions such as, inhibitory control, working memory, cognitive flexibility, planning, and decision-making [14, 15], that determines dramatically the success of individual daily living functioning, a growing interest in this concept have been emerged in the area of addictive behaviours. The negative effect of heroin use on executive functions is consistent across studies [16, 17]. Different investigations reported that heroin consumption impacts on decision-making, problem-solving, working memory [11, 12, 18], and inhibitory control [19], which reflects in impulsivity. When compared with controls, heroin-dependent subjects show higher impulsivity and more disadvantageous decisions. According to Verdejo-Garcia and Bechara [20], these subjects are also characterized by a failure to learn from mistakes and a difficulty to anticipate the consequences of their decisions.

According to these authors, patients with drug addiction are similar to patients with ventromedial prefrontal cortex lesions [21] regarding their decision-making processes

In this sense, based on the somatic-marker hypothesis originally proposed by Damasio [22], these authors presented a somatic-marker theory of addiction. This theory states that the hyperactivity in amygdala, and the hypoactivity in the prefrontal cortex could explain dysfunction in somatic markers (i.e., emotional signs). The hyperactivity of the amygdala, will generate an increased response to obtain immediate reward through the drugs. On the other hand, the hypoactivity in the prefrontal cortex may explain the difficulty to anticipate the long-term consequence of a decision. Taken together, these conditions will promote the immediate rewarding effect of heroin consumption, increasing the vulnerability of these subjects for drug abuse.

A more recent study [23], stated that patients with substance use disorder report higher level of frontal symptoms and more subjective memory complaints than non-clinical subjects. Although abstinence by itself has a positive impact on behaviours, therapeutic techniques that help in recovering emotional and cognitive processes are commonly used to help patients with substance use disorder in regaining control over their life [24]. Cognitive and emotional restructuring techniques during the post-consumption stage underlie programs to recover emotional and cognitive status, complementing opioid substitution treatment (usually with methadone), typically in the context of residential programs or community treatments [25, 26].

1.2   Traditional and ICT-Based Cognitive Training

Additionally, or complementarily to the therapeutic intervention, cognitive training programs boost the cognitive effects of the overall treatment on people with substance abuse [27]. These programs have the aim of facilitating the intervention by improving general cognitive functioning, in particular executive functioning. Conventional protocols for cognitive training include a set of techniques designed to improve particular cognitive functions [28] and enhance functionality and the capacity of individuals to live independently [29]. We believe that the generalization of the outcomes from cognitive training sessions to daily living environment would benefit from exercises that involve daily life activities. Unlike traditional treatment programs, however, we propose an intervention that reproduces in a virtual scenario the activities that people would usually do in their daily life. This approach relies on the principles of cognitive behavioural therapies, by focusing on skills acquisition, training, and generalization of acquired skills to the natural environment. It is also important to consider that this type of intervention provides greater access to treatment and the possibility of self-application.

One strategy to deliver cognitive training programs is to wrap them up as serious games [30]. Despite being designed for purposes other than entertainment, serious games retain the fundamental characteristics of games: they are interactive, provide feedback, and are appealing to the eye, and are therefore more motivating patients than non-game-like exercises. Serious games are currently used to treat several mental disorders [31] and to rehabilitate a myriad of neurological deficits and motor impairments [32].

Mobile devices, with their ever-increasing processing and interaction capabilities, are currently replacing desktops and even laptops as the main tool of work and leisure.

The growing availability of health mobile technologies – specifically designed to leverage the potential of mobile devices to manage health information, behaviours, and interactions – is broadening the accessibility of health services both to previously excluded sectors of the population and to situations for which people did not have the habit of using the health services. A further advantage of mobile technology is that the intuitiveness of the touchscreen-based interaction that comes with it facilitates usability compared to traditional PCs.

Accordingly, the development and testing of interventions based on this technology with diverse clinical samples is clearly needed. The current study tests the efficacy in a sample of patients recovering from heroin abuse of a cognitive intervention we developed using mobile technology enriched with a variety of interactive serious games.

2 Method

2.1 Participants

Patients diagnosed with substance use disorder for heroin according to the DSM-V (APA, 2013) criteria were recruited from a therapeutic community for drug dependence treatment in Portugal. The inclusion criteria were: being diagnosed with substance use disorder with an age equal to or higher than 18 years. The exclusion criteria were (1) having a diagnosis of a previous psychiatric or neurological disorders, (2) having scores below the cut-off values for their age on the Mini Mental Examination Test - MMSE [33]. One of the potential participants was excluded based on these criteria. The latter control was important because anxious systems can indicate independent sources of cognitive dysfunction [34].

Preliminary screening was performed to exclude patients who were unable or unwilling to consent to participate, including those who tested positive for metabolites of heroin, cocaine, cannabis or benzodiazepines in urine toxicology testing.

The final sample comprised 14 men undergoing methadone maintenance, with an average age of 37 years (SD = 4.48). Most of them had Secondary education (n = 10) and were single (n = 11). As for drug related variables, patients had been involved in drug abuse on average for 19 years (SD = 3.22) and most had a history of intra-venous consumption (n = 10). The great majority (n = 12) were also involved in prior treatments for drug dependence. A minority tested positive for HIV (n = 4).

2.2 Measures

The neuropsychological assessment included the two screening measures - MMSE [33] and the SCL-90-R [35] - along with the outcome measures. The outcome measures were based on known cognitive tests as well as a depression scale to assess the change in depression between the baseline and the follow-up assessment.

MMSE [33] was used to evaluate the cognitive condition and mental impairment. It consists of 30 items that measure six cognitive capacities: orientation, memory, attention and calculation, language and construct ability. Total possible scores range from 0 to 30 but cut-off scores were defined according to educational level of participant.

SCL-90-R [35] was used to measure psychological distress. It is a self-report questionnaire composed by 90 items that evaluates nine primary symptom dimensions (somatization, obsessive-compulsive, interpersonal sensitivity, depression, anxiety, hostility, phobic anxiety paranoid ideation, and psychoticism). Items are rating according a five points Likert scale ranging from "not at all" to "extremely". Global indices of general severity index, positive symptoms distress index and positive symptoms total provide information for assessment of psychological status.

Frontal Assessment Battery - FAB [36] is a useful tool for the evaluation of the integrity of the frontal lobe functions. It is composed by six subtests that evaluates six different domains of frontal functioning, namely conceptualization, mental flexibility, motor programming, sensitivity to interference, inhibitory control, and environmental autonomy. Total scores range from 0 to 18 and higher scores indicated better frontal lobe functioning.

Verbal fluency tasks. Verbal fluency was assessed with three tasks: (1) the semantic verbal fluency task (SVF); (2) action verbal fluency task (AVF); and (3) phonologic verbal fluency task (PVF). During each task participants are required to produce as many words as possible describing, respectively, animals, verb actions and words beginning with the letter "P" in one minute. The scores are calculated separately for each test by the sum of correct responses on each [37].

Rey Auditory-Verbal Learning Test – RAVLT [38]. It was used to evaluate declarative verbal memory. The RALVT consists of different word lists (each containing 15 words) that are listened by participants. The outcomes of this test were based on immediate word recall and delayed word recall (after 30 min).

Toulouse Pieron Test's - TPT [39] and the Color Trails Test's - CTT [40]. These tests were used to evaluate sustained attention. The TPT is a traditional cancelation paper and pencil test assessing attention/concentration. The task consists to identify exemplars of three targets, which are randomly presented within a set of similar figures during ten minutes. The working efficiency and dispersion indexes are used as outcomes measures.

The CTT consists of two parts: Color Trails I (CTTI) and Color Trails II (CTTII). The first trail has 25 numbers presented in yellow and ink circles and participants must connect numbers in an ascending order as quickly as possible. The trail II it is composed by 49 numbers presented in yellow and pink circles and participant is invited to connect numbers in an ascending order too, but an alternation between two different sets of stimuli (numbers and colours) is required. Performance was scored by the number of errors and execution times in trials I and II.

Wisconsin Card Sorting Test - WCST [41] was used to evaluate mental flexibility. It consists of four cards and 128 cards that vary in terms of colour, form and number. Participant must derive the correct card sorting principle using the information transmitted by the examiner. The sorting principle changes without warning after 10 consecutive correct responses. The tests ends when six categories/trails were achieved or the 128 cards were used. As outcome measures, we used the number of completed trials, correct responses, and perseverative responses.

Iowa Gambling Task's - IGT [42]. It was used in the evaluation of decision-making. In this computerized task, the goal is to win as much money as possible by choosing decks of cards. Four decks are available, however, based in losses or gains of money, some of them are bad options and others are good options. In our study the card picking strategy on advantageous and disadvantageous decks were defined as outcome measures.

Beck Depression Inventory - BDI-II [43] was also used to determine depression levels. It consists of 21 items that evaluate 21 clinical expressions of depression. Participants must rate these symptoms in terms of intensity. Total scores range from 0 to 63, with higher scores indicated severe depression. The cut-off score of 10, that indicates none of minimal depression, was used in this study.

2.3 Procedure

An ethics committee approved the study, and all participants signed an informed consent and were informed about the study prior to participation.

The patients were distributed to two different groups: the active group consisting of mHealth approach with serious games-based cognitive intervention (n = 11) and the control group consisting of methadone maintenance treatment for heroin dependence (n = 3).

The intervention consisted of 10 60-minute sessions of cognitive training with mobile technology using serious games (two to three sessions per week over the usual 4–6 week period of treatment for substance abuse). The executive training exercises performed by participants were selected in order to develop cognitive abilities related to executive functioning. In each session we sought to train more than one cognitive function in order to balance training across cognitive domains. Each session started with a brief training period, in which participants were able to (re)acquire interaction skills and familiarization with the touchscreen devices. Participants failing to complete training sessions at the beginning of the protocol were dropped and their data was not analysed. Participants accessed the exercises freely over the Internet, and their responses were registered using the device's input from the touchscreen. Therapists from the research and intervention team were involved in all stages of the study involving the participants - recruitment, assessment, and cognitive training - interacting face-to-face with them. These therapists were introduced to patients by in-house therapists, and asked patients to participate in the study, explaining its benefits, duration, and demands on patients' time and commitment. In the assessments, therapists provided, explained, and collected the assessment forms. In the cognitive simulation sessions, therapists provided the mobile devices, started the exercises, and explained how they worked to participants.

The mobile cognitive training program consisted of several mobile applications running on Android OS (Fig. 1) that were developed according to the principles of conventional neuropsychological tests in each of these cognitive areas, but with game-like features, which facilitate playfulness and motivation [31]. Some of these exercises are described elsewhere in greater detail [44]. In the last session, the same neuropsychological tests used in the first assessment were again applied.

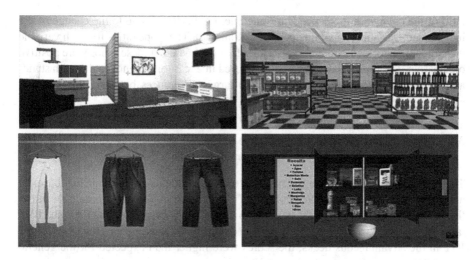

Fig. 1. Examples of the tasks used as cognitive exercises. Apartment that included some of the tasks (TOP-LEFT), Shopping task (TOP-RIGHT), Wardrobe task (BOTTOM-LEFT), Virtual kitchen task (BOTTOM-RIGHT).

The applications were installed on Samsung Galaxy 10.1" tablets. The applications used were developed using Unity 2.5 (Unity Technologies TM), and their alpha and beta versions had been previously tested by a group of students from the host institution.

3   Results

The statistical analysis started with descriptive statistics to understand whether the scores in the neuropsychological tests at baseline and follow-up assessments were below the normative data available for the general population. This analysis was done for the tests more associated with frontal brain functioning such as the FAB, PVF and the IGT tests.

Considering the discrepancy of group sizes, inferential statistics were applied only to compare the baseline assessment with the follow-up assessment. Considering this limitation, our main goal was not to determine the effects of cognitive intervention with serious games in neuropsychological adjustment, which have already showed positive effects on other populations in treatment for substance use disorders, namely alcohol use disorder [44], but to understand what are the main outcomes that should be expected in patients undergoing methadone maintenance and how the cognitive changes between assessments explain the improvement in the main outcome (frontal lobe functioning through the FAB). Thus, the data analysis started with a paired-samples t-test to determine improvements at the follow-up assessment for all the cognitive dimensions studied, including frontal lobe functions. The cognitive domains that improved with treatment were further explored by analysing the slope lines between the FAB (main outcome) and the cognitive domains in we found significant differences between pre- and post-program. The calculation of the slope between two variables allows determining the ratio of the change in the dependent (outcome, i.e. FAB) relative to the change of the independent variable (remaining cognitive domains). The slope ratios for each variable were then transformed into binary variables to reflect whether these ratios were positive or negative. The binary variables were then used in 2×2 contingency tables with standardized residuals to identify the cells with larger differences between observed and expected proportions.

3.1 Comparisons Between Performance in the Neuropsychological Tests at Baseline and Follow-up with Normative Data

The comparisons between the normative scores and patients' performance at baseline and follow-up in the FAB, PVF and the IGT are shown in Table 1. These data shows that despite the increase from the baseline to follow-up assessment in the FAB and PVF task, these scores were below the normative data at both assessments. However, for the IGT in the advantageous decks, the scores were higher than expected for the general population.

Table 1. Comparisons between performance in the neuropsychological tests with normative data

	Baseline(1)		Follow-up(2)			
	M	SD	M	SD	μ	Comparison
FAB[1]	16.14	1.75	17.50	0.76	15	$1, 2 < \mu$
PVF[2]	10.79	4.35	13.29	4.39	20	$1, 2 < \mu$
IGT deck C[3]	22.25	7.83	32.50	11.13	22	$1, 2 > \mu$
IGT deck D[3]	28.92	9.28	35.75	15.77	25	$1, 2 > \mu$

Note: FAB – Frontal Assessment Battery; PVF – Phonological Verbal Fluency; IGT – Iowa Gambling Task (Decks C and D). (1) Dubois et al. (2000) [36]; (2) Esteves et al. (2015) [45]; (3) Fernie e Tunney (2006) [46].

3.2 Comparisons Between the Baseline and the Follow-up Assessments

The paired samples t-tests were conducted on the total sample for the variables from the neuropsychological assessment. This analysis showed statistically significant improvements on the following variables, as depicted in Table 2: frontal lobe functions ($t(13) = -2.665$; $p = .019$); verbal memory in the RAVLT for both immediate ($t(13) = -4.409$; $p = .001$) and delayed verbal free recall ($t(13) = -3.257$; $p = .006$); sustained attention according to execution time in the first trial of the CTT ($t(13) = 2.175$; $p = .049$), working efficiency ($t(12) = -3.073$; $p = .010$) and dispersion index of the TPT ($t(12) = 2.306$; $p = .040$); cognitive flexibility based on the number of trials in the WCST ($t(13) = 5.186$; $p = .001$) and number of perseverative responses also in the WCST ($t(13) = 2.634$; $p = .021$); advantageous card picks (deck C) in the IGT ($t(11) = -4.611$; $p = .001$), and depression as measured by the BDI ($t(12) = 3.461$; $p = . 005$). No significant differences were found for the remaining variables (all p's $> .05$).

Table 2. Comparisons between baseline and follow-up assessments for neuropsychological measures

	Baseline		Follow-up		
	M	SD	M	SD	t
FAB	16.14	1.75	17.50	0.76	−2.665*
RAVLT IR	35.00	11.54	46.79	11.10	−4.409**
RAVLT DR	7.79	4.35	10.36	3.41	−3.257**
SVF	17.50	5.65	18.43	4.82	−0.671
AVF	10.57	4.22	12.36	4.55	−1.623
PVF	10.79	4.35	13.29	4.39	−1.836
CTT-I errors	0.86	1.03	0.21	0.43	2.175*
CTT-I ET	53.36	28.68	39.79	19.01	1.883
CTT-II errors	1.07	1.27	0.29	0.61	1.844
CTT-II ET	101.57	61.36	75.79	26.10	1.863
TPT WE	135.23	70.75	167.46	81.63	−3.073*
TPT DI	28.88	30.34	19.43	24.37	2.306*
WCST trials	113.29	17.47	84.21	20.58	5.186***
WCST hits	70.36	10.46	63.36	16.81	1.242
WCST P	25.57	21.50	11.50	15.65	2.634*
IGT deck C	22.25	7.83	32.50	11.13	−4.611**
IGT deck D	28.92	9.28	35.75	15.77	−1.507
BDI	24.85	16.06	14.00	13.64	3.461**

Note: $* p < .05; ** p < .01; *** p < .001$.

FAB – Frontal Assessment Battery; RAVLT IR – Rey Auditory-Verbal Learning Test immediate word recall; RAVLT - Rey Auditory-Verbal Learning Test delayed word recall; SVF – Semantic Verbal Fluency; AVF – Action Verbal Fluency; PVF – Phonologic Verbal Fluency; CTT errors – number of errors on the Color Trails Test; CTT ET – execution time on the Color Trails Test; TPT WE – working efficiency of the Toulouse Pieron Test; TPT DI – dispersion index of the Toulouse Pieron Test; WCST trials – number of trials of the Wisconsin Card Sorting Test; WCST hits – correct responses of the Wisconsin Card Sorting Test; WCST P – perseverative responses of the Wisconsin Card Sorting Test; IGT – Iowa Gambling Task; BDI – Beck Depression Inventory.

3.3 Linear Change Between Assessments

The rate of change in the FAB total score (Y) as a function of rates of changes in each of the independent variables (X) was calculated with the use of slope lines. The slope lines were calculated for variables with significant differences between times 1 and 2 only. The slope (m) for each variable was calculated according to the following expression: $m = \Delta Y/\Delta X \iff m = Y2–Y1/X2–X1$, in which Y denotes the dependent variable and X the independent variable. The m is positive if the dependent variable changes in the same direction of the independent variable, whereas a negative score describes the opposite. These variables were then coded into binary variables as being a positive outcome (1) or a negative outcome (0). Following this procedure, 2 × 2 contingency tables with adjusted standardised residuals (ASRs) were calculated with group (active vs. controls) for columns and each of these binary variables for rows.

This analysis showed that differences between observed and expected proportions were larger for delayed word recall of the RAVLT and for the number of perseverative responses of the WCST. This suggests that the proportions of positive outcomes were higher in the active group (ASRs = 1.7) than in the controls (ASRs = −1.7) in the delayed word recall of the RAVLT (Table 3) as well as for the number of perseverative responses of the WCST (active group ASRs = 1.6 vs. controls ASRs = −1.6) in Table 4.

Table 3. Contingency 2 × 2 table for group (active vs. controls) by the outcome on delayed word recall of the Rey Auditory-Verbal Learning Test

		Active group	Controls	Total
Negative outcome	Count	3	2	5
	Adjusted Residual	−1.7	1.7	
Positive outcome	Count	6	0	6
	Adjusted Residual	1.7	−1.7	
Total	Count	9	2	11

Table 4. Contingency 2 × 2 table for group (active vs. controls) by the outcome on perseverative responses of the Wisconsin Card Sorting Test

		Active group	Controls	Total
Negative outcome	Count	2	2	4
	Adjusted Residual	−1.6	1.6	
Positive outcome	Count	9	1	10
	Adjusted Residual	1.6	−1.6	
Total	Count	11	3	14

4 Discussion

The main objective of this study was to explore the efficacy of a SG-based cognitive training program in patients undergoing methadone maintenance. We were also interested in exploring how the cognitive changes between baseline and follow-up assessments explain the improvement in frontal lobe functioning after treatment. The impact of heroin consumption on the frontal lobes [6–8] and executive functions [11–13, 16–18] is well reported in the literature. It is similar to the impact of alcohol use disorder [44], for which cognitive stimulation using serious games has been found to contribute significantly to cognitive recovery in patients undergoing rehabilitation [43].

Our results indicate a consistent improvement in cognitive functioning between baseline and follow-up assessment in terms of frontal lobe functions, verbal memory and sustained attention, as well as in some aspects of cognitive flexibility and decision-making. Depression levels also improved between baseline and follow-up. However, the discrepancy of group sizes and very small size of the control group did not allow us to use inferential statistics to determine whether these differences change across groups. To help understanding these improvements, we instead analysed the slope to determine how the change in each cognitive domain relates with the change in frontal lobe functioning. The analysis of the frequency of positive outcomes (i.e. positive change in the independent variable as in the main outcome) and negative outcomes (i.e. negative change in the independent variable in an opposite direction to the main outcome) showed that higher proportions of positive outcomes were expected for controls in both verbal memory through delayed recall ability and in cognitive flexibility through one of the indicators of the WCST. Nevertheless, these results should be interpreted with caution given the small sample used in this study.

Overall, our results indicate that the negative effects of heroin abuse on the frontal lobes may be attenuated by treatment, but it was not possible to ascertain the specific effects of cognitive intervention on the global improvement at the follow-up. Larger-scale clinical trials with heroin patients are required for this.

Together with the assessment of the contribution of SG-based treatments to patients' improvement at the cognitive level, future research should also focus on motivational gains in the use of such computer-based solutions, and its possible influence on the effectiveness of the treatment. It would also be important to compare patients enrolled in traditional cognitive rehabilitation programs with patients in mixed rehabilitation programs, in order to identify the magnitude of the therapeutic gain that this technique may offer. Another issue that needs to be addressed is the cost-benefit advantages of these programs: between two equally effective programs, one that provides the same treatment effects at lower cost will be considered advantageous for mental health care.

Acknowledgments. The authors would like to thank to the clinical staff of Ares do Pinhal that participated in patients' recruitment and data collection.

References

1. UNODC. World Drug Report 2013. United Nations publication (2012). e-ISBN: 978-92-1-055653-8
2. NSDUH. National Survey on Drug Use and Health 2012. Substance Abuse and Mental Health Data Archive (SAMHDA) (2012). http://doi.org/10.3886/ICPSR34933.v2
3. Oldendorf, W.H., Hyman, S., Braun, L., Oldendorf, S.Z.: Blood-brain barrier: penetration of morphine, codeine, heroin, and methadone after carotid injection. Science **178**(4064), 984–986 (1972)
4. Sawynok, J.: The therapeutic use of heroin: a review of the pharmacological literature. Can. J. Physiol. Pharmacol. **64**(1), 1–6 (1986)
5. Stahl, S.M.: Essential Psychopharmacology: Neuroscientific Basis and Practical Applications. Cambridge University Press, Cambridge (2008)

6. Schmidt, A., Borgwardt, S., Gerber, H., Wiesbeck, G.A., Schmid, O., Riecher-Rössler, A., Smieskova, R., Lang, U.E., Walter, M.: Acute effects of heroin on negative emotional processing: relation of amygdala activity and stress-related responses. Biol. Psychiatry **76**(4), 289–296 (2014)
7. Cheng, G.L.F., Zeng, H., Leung, M.K., Zhang, H.-J., Lau, B.M.W., Liu, Y.-P., et al.: Heroin abuse accelerates biological aging: a novel insight from telomerase and brain imaging interaction. Trans. Psychiatry **3**, e260 (2013). doi:10.1038/tp.2013.36
8. Goldstein, R.Z., Volkow, N.D.: Dysfunction of the prefrontal cortex in addiction: neuroimaging findings and clinical implication. Nat. Rev. Neurosci. **12**(11), 652–669 (2011). doi:10.1038/nrn3119
9. Fuster, J.: Frontal lobe and cognitive development. J. Neurosychol. **31**, 373–385 (2002)
10. Stuss, D.T., Levine, B.: Adult Clinical Neuropsychology: Lessons from studies of the frontal lobes. Ann. Rev. Psychol. **53**, 401–433 (2002)
11. Ersche, K.D., Clark, L., London, M., Robbins, T.W., Sahakian, B.J.: Profile of executive and memory function associated with amphetamine and opiate dependence. Neuropsychopharmacology **31**(5), 1036–1047 (2006)
12. Pirastu, M., Fais, R., Messina, M., Bini, V., Spiga, S., Falconieri, D., Diana, M.: Impaired decision-making in opiate-dependent subjects: effect of pharmacological therapies. Drug Alcohol. Depend. **83**, 163–168 (2006)
13. Gurber, S.A., Silveri, M.M., Yurgelun-Todd, D.A.: Neuropsychological consequences of opiate use. Neuropsychol. Rev. **17**, 299–315 (2007). doi:10.1007/s11065-007-9041-y
14. Miyake, A., Friedman, N.P., Emerson, M., Witzki, X., Howerter, A.: The unity and diversity of executive functions and their contributions to complex "Frontal Lobe" tasks: A latent variable analysis. Cog. Psychol. **41**, 49–100 (2000). doi:10.1006/cogp.1999.0734
15. Verdejo, A.G., Bechara, A.: Neuropsicologia de las funciones ejecutivas. Psicoth **22**(2), 227–235 (2010)
16. Brand, M., Roth-Bauer, M., Driessen, M., Markowitsch, H.J.: Executive functions and risky decision-making in patients with opiate dependence. Drug Alcohol. Depend. **97**(1–2), 64–72 (2008)
17. Al-Zahrani, M.A., Elsayed, Y.A.: The impacts of substance abuse and dependence on neuropsychological functions in a simple of patients from Saudi Arabia. Behav. Brain Functions **5**, 48 (2009). doi:10.1186/1744-9081-5-48
18. Fishbeina, D.H., Krupitskyb, E., Flannerya, B.A., Langevinc, D.J., Bobashevd, G., Verbitskaya, E., et al.: Neurocognitive characterizations of Russian heroin addicts without a significant history of other drug use. Drug Alcohol Depend. **90**(1), 25–38 (2007)
19. Vassileva, J., Georgiev, S., Martin, E., Gonzalez, R., Segala, L.: Psychopathic heroin addicts are not uniformly impaired across neurocognitive domains of impulsivity. Drug Alcohol Depend. **114**(2–3), 194–200 (2011). doi:10.1016/j.drugalcdep.2010.09.021
20. Verdejo-Garcia, A., Bechara, A.: A somatic-marker theory of addiction. Neuropharmacology **56**(Suppl. 1), 48–62 (2009). doi:10.1016/j.neuropharm.2008.07.035
21. Bechara, A., Tranel, D., Damasio, H.: Characterization of the decision-making deficit of patients with ventromedial prefrontal cortex lesions. Brain **123**, 2189–2202 (2000)
22. Damasio, A.R.: Descartes' Error: Emotion, Reason, and the Human Brain. Grosset/Putnam, New York (1994)
23. Terán-Mendoza, O., Sira-Ramos, D., Guerrero-Alcedo, J., Arroyo-Alvarado, D.: Sintomatología frontal, estrés autopercibido y quejas subjetivas de memoria en adictos a sustancias. Revista de Neurología **62**, 296–302 (2016)
24. Heather, N., Greeley, J.: Cue exposure in the treatment of drug dependence: the potential of a new method for preventing relapse. Drug Alcohol. Rev. **9**(2), 155–168 (1990)

25. Passetti, F., Clark, L., Mehta, M.A., Joyce, E., King, M.: Neuropsychological predictors of clinical outcome in opiate addiction. Drug Alcohol. Depend. **94**, 82–91 (2008)
26. Rezapour, T., Hatami, J., Farhoudian, A., Sofuoglu, M., Noroozi, A., Daneshmand, R., et al.: NEuro COgnitive REhabilitation for Disease of Addiction (NECOREDA) Program: From Development to Trial. Basic Clin. Neurosci. **6**(4), 291–298 (2015)
27. Ruiz-Sánchez de León, J.M., Pedrero-Pérez, E.J., Rojo-Mota, G., Llanero-Luque, M., Puerta-García, C.: A proposal for a protocol of neuropsychological assessment for use in addictions. Rev. Neurol. **53**(8), 483–493 (2011)
28. Clare, L., Woods, R.T.: Cognitive Training and Cognitive Rehabilitation for people with early-stage Alzheimer's disease: a review. Neuropsychological Rehabil. **14**, 385–401 (2004)
29. Willis, S.L., Tennstedt, S.L., Marsiske, M., Ball, K., Elias, J., Koepke, K.M., Morris, J.N., Rebok, G.W., Unverzagt, F.W., Stoddard, A.M., Wright, E., ACTIVE Study Group: Long-term effects of cognitive training on everyday functional outcomes in older adults. JAMA **296**(23), 2805–2814 (2006)
30. Lange, B., Requejo, P., Flynn, S., Rizzo, A., Valero-Cuevas, F., Baker, L., Winstein, C.: The potential of virtual reality and gaming to assist successful aging with disability. Phys. Med. Rehabil. Clin. N Am. **21**(2), 339–356 (2010)
31. Gamito, P., Oliveira, J., Morais, D., Rosa, P., Saraiva, T.: Serious games for serious problems: from ludicus to therapeuticus. In: Kim, J.J. (ed.) Virtual Reality, pp. 527–548. InTech Publishing (2011)
32. Gamito, P., Oliveira, J., Morais, D., Rosa, P., Saraiva, T.: NeuAR – a look into AR applications in the neurosciences area. In: Nee, A., Ong, S. (eds.) Augmented Reality. INTECH, pp. 131–154 (2011)
33. Folstein, M.F., Folstein, S.E., McHugh, P.R.: Mini-mental state: a practical method for grading the cognitive state of patients for the clinician. J. Psychiatr. Res. **12**, 189–198 (1975)
34. Stillman, A.N., Rowe, K.C., Arndt, S., Moser, D.J.: Anxious symptoms and cognitive function in non-demented older adults: an inverse relationship. Int. J. Geriatric Psychiatry **27**(8), 792–798 (2012)
35. Derogatis, L.R., Savitz, K.L.: The SCL-90-R and the Brief Symptom Inventory (BSI) in Primary Care. In: Maruish, M.E. (ed.) Handbook of Psychological Assessment in Primary Care Setting, vol. 236, pp. 297–334. Laurence Erlbaum Associates, Mahwah (2000)
36. Dubois, B., Slachevsky, A., Litvan, I., Pillon, B.: The FAB: a frontal assessment battery at bedside. Neurology **55**, 1621–1626 (2000)
37. Brucki, D., Makheiros, S., Okamoto, I., Bertolucci, P.: Dados normativos para o teste de fluência verbal categoria animais em nosso meio. (Normative data: category verbal fluency). Arquivos de Neuro-Psiquiatra **55**(1), 56–61 (1997)
38. Rey, A.: L'examen clinique en psychologie (The psychological examination). Presses Universitaires de France, Paris (1958)
39. Toulouse, E., Pieron, H.: Prueba perceptiva y de atención. Tea Ediciones, Madrid, Spain (1986)
40. D'Elia, L., Satz, P., Uchiyama, C., White, T.: Color trails test professional manual. Psychological Assessment Resources, Odessa, FL (1996)
41. Heaton, R.K., Chelune, G.J., Talley, J.L., Kay, G.G., Curtiss, G.: Wisconsin card sorting test (WCST) — manual revised and expanded. Psychological Assessment Resources, Odessa (1993)
42. Bechara, A., Damásio, A.R., Damásio, H., Anderson, S.W.: Insensitivity to future consequences following damage to human prefrontal cortex. Cognition **50**(1–3), 7–15 (1994)
43. Beck, A.T., Steer, R.A., Brown, G.K.: BDI-II: Beck Depression Inventory Manual. Psychological Corporation, San Antonio (1996)

44. Gamito, P., Oliveira, J., Lopes, P., Brito, R., Morais, D., Silva, D., Silva, A., Rebelo, S., Bastos, M., Deus, A.: Executive functioning in alcoholics following an mHealth cognitive stimulation program: randomized controlled trial. J. Med. Internet Res. **16**(4), e102 (2014)
45. Esteves, C.S., Oliveira, C.R., Moret-Tatay, C., Navarro-Pardo, E., De Carlia, G.A., Silva, I.G., et al.: honemic and semantic verbal fluency tasks: normative data for elderly Brazilians. Psychology/Psicologia Reflexão e Crítica **28**(2), 350–355 (2015)
46. Fernie, G., Tunney, R.J.: Some decks are better than others: The effect of reinforcer type and task instructions on learning in the Iowa gambling task. Brain Cogn. **60**, 94–102 (2006)

Intuitively Evaluating Balance Measurement Software Using Kinect2

Zhihan Lv$^{(\boxtimes)}$, Vicente Penades, Sonia Blasco, Javier Chirivella,
and Pablo Gagliardo

FIVAN, Valencia, Spain
lvzhihan@gmail.com

Abstract. A balance measurement software based on Kinect2 sensor
is evaluated by comparing to golden standard balance measure platform
intuitively. The software analysis the tracked body data from the user by
Kinect2 sensor and get user's center of mass (CoM) as well as its motion
route on a plane. The software is evaluated by several comparison tests,
the evaluation results preliminarily prove the reliability of the software.

Keywords: Virtual reality · Center of mass · Balance measurement

1 Introduction

Nowadays, there are many software and hardware approaches for human balance measurement, include various of hardware based balance measurement device [2,4,6,7,15,21,37,40,42], Kinect based device [3,11,12,16,38], sensor network based device [19,39,44], hybrid device [36], evaluation investigation [13,14], related interaction technology [1,9,10]. This work is the extension version of our work on Rehab2015 [34].

The evaluated software employs distinctive calculation approach of mass of center. The center of mass is the quality of the object balance. If a pivot is placed at this point, the object will remain in place, and balance. The center of mass of a system is not always in the geometric center of the system. When a system is built around its center of mass balance, it is considered to be in equilibrium. The center of mass can be called a pivot point in which the system can rotate around it. The system revolves around the force of a rotational equivalent, called a torque, which rotates the system clockwise or counterclockwise. The balance in the system is the result of a system in which the center of mass is placed with a pivot and has a zero net torque. Long, on each end of the rigid body, the torque is a torque on one end and the other end is equal in magnitude, but opposite in direction, the net torque generated zero. The calculation process for each frame includes three steps. First, pre-processing step filters the noises from the range images and further removes the obstacles in the view. As shown in Fig. 2 up, the obstacles are marked in red color to warn the players to clean them for safety measurement, meanwhile, the obstacles are removed from the system memory

© Springer International Publishing AG 2017
H.M. Fardoun et al. (Eds.): REHAB 2015, CCIS 665, pp. 83–93, 2017.
https://doi.org/10.1007/978-3-319-69694-2_8

so that the software can focus on calculating the valid data. In the second step, the center of mass (CoM) of the user is calculated according to the CoM of every part of user's body, as well as considering the weights of all parts. Finally, the CoM is mapped to a plane and recorded to the cloud based sever located in our headquarter. In the detection of the human body, to use the bone identification. A general method for skeletal identification is a learning system to transfer each the segmentation pixel of the human body images to identify the body parts of the movement capture device, the system finally output a particular pixel that belongs to which parts of the body. Skeletal identification mixed the anthropometry and gait recognition science, physiological characteristics and behavior characteristics of the comprehensive human identification. Skeleton recognition system is the first to extract the body's static skeleton information through the Kinect camera skeleton tracking function. Then it uses the joint angle of the legs or 3D to describe the gait characteristics. Finally, according to the results to complete the identification. The information is limited which produced by Kinect. To use Kinect to create a real sense of fun and memorable applications, it also need some other information. This is the original intention of bone tracking technology. Bone tracking technique is used to establish the coordinate of each joint point of the human body through depth data, and to determine the important information of the joint point. Bone tracking can determine the main part of the human body, such as the recognition of the head and hands, etc. Skeletal tracking technique is determined by the depth data generated by Kinect. Skeleton tracking system uses the depth of field of the image processing technology and use more complex algorithms such as matrix transform, machine learning and other methods to determine skeletal coordinates. Kinect can track up to 25 bone nodes, the current Kinect can only track the human body. For other objects, it cannot realize. Joint points of the human body recognition is single input depth image which segmented into dense probability body component tags, components definition is related bone joint space similar parts of the body. The recognition of human joint points can be divided into three steps: (1) Remove the background, the use of distance sensor analysis to find the most probable region of the human body, through the edge detection to determine the edge of the target area, and to achieve the segmentation of the human body contour. (2) Body parts recognition. It mainly identifies various parts of the body, such as the head, limbs, trunk and so on. (3) Recognition of joint points of human body. Human body parts are connected through joint point, Kinect from the front, side and other direction analysis of all the pixels to determine the location of the joint coordinates of points.

The Kinect2 face recognition, motion tracking, and resolution are much more precise than the Kinect1. Kinect2 uses "time of flight" technology to determine the features and motion of certain objects. IGN summarized this technology well by comparing it to sonar technology, except that this is a large improvement and more accurate. By using this technology, the Kinect2 can see just as well in a completely dark room as in a well-lit room. Although the first Kinect used similar technology, the Kinect2 has greatly improved upon it. The Kinect2 has 1080 resolution (HD), compared to the previous generation of VGA sensor is a huge improvement. Kinect2 allows a more accurate face recognition feature, which can get more clear images and video information. This clear video information will come in handy in the new Skype integration capabilities. They also increase the maximum resolution that the depth sensor can support to allow for more details, such as finger movements and limb positioning. The new Kinect Xbox data processing capacity of up to 2 GB/s. Microsoft also read the depth of the flight time calculation method to replace the existing light measurement method, making the new Kinect faster and more accurate than the original Kinect. The method is based on the most accurate time calculation method that is based on a single photon bounce back from an object or person. Kinect2 can process 2 gigabytes of data per second, USB3 provides almost 10x faster broadband for the data transfer, 60% wider field of vision, and can detect and track 20 joints from 6 people's bodies including thumbs. In comparison, the Kinect1 could only track 20 joints from 2 people. On top of this, when using Kinect2 we are capable of detecting heart rates, facial expressions and weights on limbs, along with much more extremely valuable biometric data. The Kinect 1.0 device doesn't have the fidelity to individually track fingers and stretching and shrinking with hands and arms but the Kinect2 has these capabilities. It's clear that this technology is certainly much more powerful and complex than the first generation of Kinect.

The recommended minimum distance from Kinect 2 for full body tracking is 4.5 ft, which is equal to 137.16 cm. In our system, we set the distance as 180–200 cm.

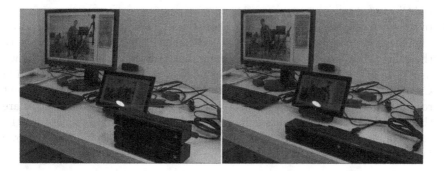

Fig. 1. Left: Place two kinect2 side by side longitudinally; Right: Place two kinect2 side by side laterally.

2 Evaluation

Three comparison tests are conducted to evaluate the performance of the software.

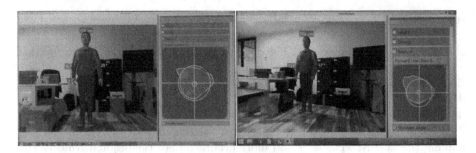

Fig. 2. The real-time balance measurement comparison results from evaluation 2. (Color figure online)

1. The first test is to check whether the tiny offset of the kinect can affect the estimated CoM value. We compared the results of two kinects with tiny longitudinal or lateral offset, as shown in Fig. 1. The comparison results indicate that there isn't significant difference. Especially, the kinects with longitudinal offset got very similar balance measurement results.
2. The purpose of the second test is to evaluate how heavy can the error of estimation result reach when the kinects have far lateral offset. We compared the results of two kinects with far lateral offset and the same target point, as shown in Fig. 3. The results indicate the visually recognizable difference of the results from two kinects, but they are still acceptable results for our application scenarios. The results are shown as in the blue window on the right in Fig. 3 up.
3. In the third test, we plan to evaluate the estimated result by a known accurate reference. We compared the kinect based balance measurement software to the golden standard balance measurement platform (made by IBV), as shown in Fig. 4. IBV platform hasn't provided SDK or recorded dynamic motion of CoM, so we use unaided eye to observe and compare the balance measurement results. The results indicate that the rough regions of the center of mass are the same. IBV platform shows more sensitive performance to capture the center of mass. Conversely, kinect based balance measurement software shows more smooth results.

The evaluation results proved the reliability of the demonstrated balance measurement software.

3   Discussion

The purpose of this work is to evaluate the CoM estimation algorithm of our developed balance measurement software. The method we employed is comparing the estimated result of the software with a known golden-standard reference (IBV balance measurement platform). The evaluation proceed is fairly preliminary, since the current evaluation is based on intuitive vision feedback, but not rigorous

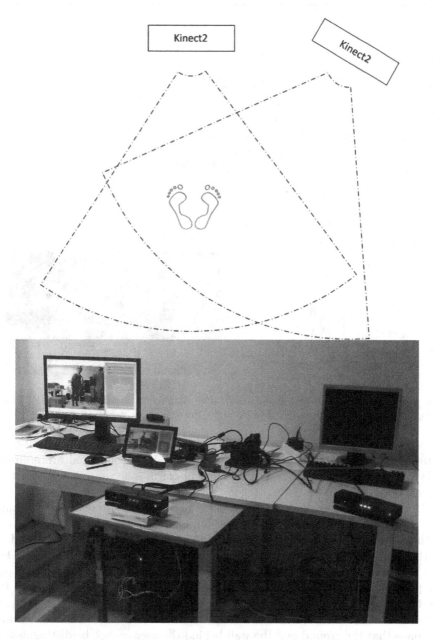

Fig. 3. Two kinects with far lateral offset and the same target point. Up: top view; Down: perspective view (Color figure online)

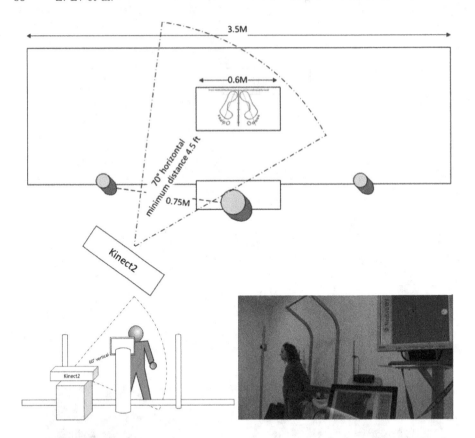

Fig. 4. Comparing the kinect based balance measurement software to the IBV plat-form. Up: top view; Bottom-left: frontal view; Bottom-right: perspective view

data analysis. However, the three evaluations we have conducted are entirely able to prove that our balance measurement platform is accurate enough for the clinical observation.

During the three evaluations, some extreme conditions are tested. For example, the estimation error caused by the minimum offset and maximum offset of the location of the kinect have been evaluated. In addition, some flaws due to the limitation of kinect hardware are detected during the evaluations. The first limitation is that the accurate rate of the estimated CoM value depends on the positional relationship between the user with kinect. When the user face to the kinect sensor, the estimation result is the most accurate since the skeleton estimated from the kinect data has the most quality in this case. The second limitation is that the ground and the wall behind the user cannot be distinguished clearly from the user's body by kinect, which causes the estimation errors. To solve this practical problem, we put some white towels on the junction between the ground and the wall, as well as the junction between the ground and the chassis of balance measurement platform, the junction between the wall and the back of the balance measurement platform.

As we mentioned before, the ultimate purposed of this research is to improve our balance measurement software. The manifested issues during the evaluations have been solved through filtering the kinect data.

4   Conclusion

The evaluations described in this paper have proved that our balance measurement software based on the CoM estimation algorithm is reliable preliminarily. The evaluations proceed also indicated some flaws of the test version. We have solved all the flaws and improved the software according to our original purpose of the evaluations. The conducted intuitive evaluation is the first step of the comprehensive evaluation of our balance measurement software, and reveals most of the existing non-core issues of the software. In next step, we plan to evaluate and further to improve the software by comparing the CoM value estimated by Wii balance board (WBB) with that by our software using numerical analysis method. Some novel technology will also be used to improve this research, e.g., Sensors [45], Virtual Rehabilitation [22,24–26,32,33], HCI [27–31,41], Video Game [5,35], Computer Vision [20,46], Database [43,50], Network and Bigdata [17,18,23,51], Optimization Algorithm [8,47–49].

Acknowledgment. The work is supported by LanPercept, a Marie Curie ITN funded through the 7th EU Framework Programme (316748).

References

1. Akbaba, Y.A., Yeldan, I., Guney, N., Ozdincler, A.R.: Intensive supervision of rehabilitation programme improves balance and functionality in the short term after bilateral total knee arthroplasty. Knee Surgery, Sports Traumatology, Arthroscopy, pp. 1–8 (2014)
2. Anson, E., Kiemel, T., Jeka, J., et al.: Visual feedback during treadmill walking improves balance for older adults: a preliminary report. In: 2013 International Conference on Virtual Rehabilitation (ICVR), pp. 166–167. IEEE (2013)
3. Biskupski, A., Fender, A.R., Feuchtner, T.M., Karsten, M., Willaredt, J.D.: Drunken ed: a balance game for public large screen displays. In: CHI 2014 Extended Abstracts on Human Factors in Computing Systems, pp. 289–292. ACM (2014)
4. Brassard, S., Otis, M.J.-D., Poirier, A., Menelas, B.-A.J.: Towards an automatic version of the berg balance scale test through a serious game. In: Proceedings of the Second ACM Workshop on Mobile Systems, Applications, and Services for Healthcare, p. 5. ACM (2012)
5. Chen, Z., Huang, W., Lv, Z.: Towards a face recognition method based on uncorrelated discriminant sparse preserving projection. Multimedia Tools Appl., 1–15 (2015)
6. Cikajlo, I., Oblak, J., Matjacic, Z.: Haptic floor for virtual balance training. In: 2011 IEEE World Haptics Conference (WHC), pp. 179–184. IEEE (2011)

7. Cikajlo, I., Rudolf, M., Goljar, N., Matjacic, Z.: Virtual reality task for telereha-bilitation dynamic balance training in stroke subjects. In: Virtual Rehabilitation International Conference, pp. 121–125. IEEE (2009)

8. Dang, S., Ju, J., Matthews, D., Feng, X., Zuo, C.: Efficient solar power heating system based on lenticular condensation. In: 2014 International Conference on Information Science, Electronics and Electrical Engineering (ISEEE), vol. 2, pp. 736–739, April 2014

9. Duh, H.B.-L., Parker, D.E., Furness, T.A.: An "independent visual background" reduced balance disturbance envoked by visual scene motion: implication for alle-viating simulator sickness. In: Proceedings of the SIGCHI Conference on Human Factors in Computing Systems, pp. 85–89. ACM (2001)

10. Ferrazzoli, D., Bera, R., Maestri, R., Perini, G., Spina, L., Gargantini, R., Pezzoli, G., Frazzitta, G.: Measuring the effectiveness of an intensive rehabilita-tion treatment on balance parameters in patients with parkinson's disease through a stabilometric platform. In: Jensen, W., Andersen, O., Akay, M. (eds.) Replace, Repair, Restore, Relieve – Bridging Clinical and Engineering Solutions in Neu-rorehabilitation. Biosystems & Biorobotics, vol. 7, pp. 369–372. Springer, Cham (2014)

11. Funaya, H., Shibata, T., Wada, Y., Yamanaka, T.: Accuracy assessment of Kinect body tracker in instant posturography for balance disorders. In: 2013 7th Inter-national Symposium on Medical Information and Communication Technology (ISMICT), pp. 213–217. IEEE (2013)

12. Garrido, J.E., Marset, I., Penichet, V.M., Lozano, M.D.: Balance disorder rehabili-tation through movement interaction. In: Proceedings of the 7th International Con-ference on Pervasive Computing Technologies for Healthcare, pp. 319–322 (2013)

13. Gil-Gómez, J.-A., Gil-Gómez, H., Lozano-Quilis, J.-A., Manzano-Hernández, P., Albiol-Pérez, S., Aula-Valero, C.: SEQ: suitability evaluation questionnaire for virtual rehabilitation systems. Application in a virtual rehabilitation system for balance rehabilitation. In: Proceedings of the 7th International Conference on Per-vasive Computing Technologies for Healthcare, pp. 335–338 (2013)

14. Hardy, S., Kern, A., Dutz, T., Weber, C., Göbel, S., Steinmetz, R.: What makes games challenging?: Considerations on how to determine the challenge posed by an exergame for balance training. In: Proceedings of the 2014 ACM International Workshop on Serious Games, pp. 57–62. ACM (2014)

15. Jacobson, J., Redfern, M.S., Furman, J.M., Whitney, S.L., Sparto, P.J., Wilson, J.B., Hodges, L.F.: Balance nave: a virtual reality facility for research and rehabil-itation of balance disorders. In: Proceedings of the ACM Symposium on Virtual Reality Software and Technology, pp. 103–109. ACM (2001)

16. Jaume-i Capo, A., Martinez-Bueso, P., Moya-Alcover, B., Varona, J.: Interactive rehabilitation system for improvement of balance therapies in people with cerebral palsy. IEEE Trans. Neural Syst. Rehabil. Eng. **22**(2), 419–427 (2014)

17. Jiang, D., Xu, Z., Lv, Z.: A multicast delivery approach with minimum energy consumption for wireless multi-hop networks. Telecommun. Syst., 1–12 (2015)

18. Jiang, D., Ying, X., Han, Y., Lv, Z.: Collaborative multi-hop routing in cognitive wireless networks. Wireless Pers. Commun., 1–23 (2015)

19. Leo, K., Tan, B.: User-tracking mobile floor projection virtual reality game system for paediatric gait & dynamic balance training. In: Proceedings of the 4th Inter-national Convention on Rehabilitation Engineering & Assistive Technology, p. 25 (2010)

20. Liu, Y., Yang, J., Meng, Q., Lv, Z., Song, Z., Gao, Z.: Stereoscopic image quality assessment method based on binocular combination saliency model. Sig. Process. **125**, 237–248 (2016)
21. Luu, B.L., Huryn, T.P., Van der Loos, H., Croft, E.A., Blouin, J.: Validation of a robotic balance system for investigations in the control of human standing balance. IEEE Trans. Neural Syst. Rehabil. Eng. **19**(4), 382–390 (2011)
22. Lv, Z.: Bringing immersive enjoyment to hyperbaric oxygen chamber users using virtual reality glasses. In: Proceedings of the 3rd 2015 Workshop on ICTs for improving Patients Rehabilitation Research Techniques, pp. 156–159. ACM (2015)
23. Lv, Z., Chirivella, J., Gagliardo, P.: Bigdata oriented multimedia mobile health applications. J. Med. Syst. **40**(5), 1–10 (2016)
24. Lv, Z., Esteve, C., Chirivella, J., Gagliardo, P.: Clinical feedback and technology selection of game based dysphonic rehabilitation tool. In: 9th International Conference on Pervasive Computing Technologies for Healthcare (PervasiveHealth2015). IEEE (2015)
25. Lv, Z., Esteve, C., Chirivella, J., Gagliardo, P.: A game based assistive tool for rehabilitation of dysphonic patients. In: 2015 3rd IEEE VR International Workshop on Virtual and Augmented Assistive Technology (VAAT), pp. 9–14, March 2015
26. Lv, Z., Esteve, C., Chirivella, J., Gagliardo, P.: Serious game based dysphonic rehabilitation tool. In: International Conference on Virtual Rehabilitation (ICVR2015). IEEE (2015)
27. Lv, Z., Feng, L., Li, H., Feng, S.: Hand-free motion interaction on Google glass. In: SIGGRAPH Asia 2014 Mobile Graphics and Interactive Applications. ACM (2014)
28. Lv, Z., Feng, S., Feng, L., Li, H.: Extending touch-less interaction on vision based wearable device. In: 2015 IEEE Virtual Reality (VR), pp. 231–232, March 2015
29. Lv, Z., Feng, S., Khan, M.S.L., Ur Réhman, S., Li, H.: Foot motion sensing: augmented game interface based on foot interaction for smartphone. In: CHI 2014 Extended Abstracts on Human Factors in Computing Systems, pp. 293–296. ACM (2014)
30. Lv, Z., Halawani, A., Feng, S., Li, H., Ur Réhman, S.: Multimodal hand and foot gesture interaction for handheld devices. ACM Trans. Multimedia Comput. Commun. Appl. (TOMM) **11**(1s), 1–19 (2014)
31. Lv, Z., Halawani, A., Feng, S., Ur Réhman, S., Li, H.: Touch-less interactive augmented reality game on vision-based wearable device. Pers. Ubiquit. Comput. **19**(3–4), 551–567 (2015)
32. Lv, Z., Li, H.: Imagining in-air interaction for hemiplegia sufferer. In: International Conference on Virtual Rehabilitation (ICVR2015). IEEE (2015)
33. Lv, Z., Penades, V., Blasco, S., Chirivella, J., Gagliardo, P.: Comparing Kinect2 based balance measurement software to Wii Balance Board. In: Proceedings of the 3rd 2015 Workshop on ICTs for Improving Patients Rehabilitation Research Techniques, pp. 50–53. ACM (2015)
34. Lv, Z., Penades, V., Blasco, S., Chirivella, J., Gagliardo, P.: Intuitive evaluation of Kinect2 based balance measurement software. In; Proceedings of the 3rd 2015 Workshop on ICTs for Improving Patients Rehabilitation Research Techniques, pp. 62–65. ACM (2015)
35. Lv, Z., Tek, A., Da Silva, F., Empereur-Mot, C., Chavent, M., Baaden, M.: Game on, science-how video game technology may help biologists tackle visualization challenges. PloS One **8**(3), 57990 (2013)

36. Muñoz, J.E., Chavarriaga, R., Lopez, D.S.: Application of hybrid BCI and exergames for balance rehabilitation after stroke. In: Proceedings of the 11th Conference on Advances in Computer Entertainment Technology, p. 67. ACM (2014)

37. Oddsson, L.I., Konrad, J., Williams, S.R., Karlsson, R., Ince, S.: A rehabilitation tool for functional balance using altered gravity and virtual reality. In: 2006 International Workshop on Virtual Rehabilitation, pp. 193–196. IEEE

38. Pisan, Y., Marin, J.G., Navarro, K.F.: Improving lives: using Microsoft Kinect to predict the loss of balance for elderly users under cognitive load. In: Proceedings of The 9th Australasian Conference on Interactive Entertainment: Matters of Life and Death, p. 29. ACM (2013)

39. Ramachandran, R., Ramanna, L., Ghasemzadeh, H., Pradhan, G., Jafari, R., Prabhakaran, B.: Body sensor networks to evaluate standing balance: interpreting muscular activities based on inertial sensors. In: Proceedings of the 2nd International Workshop on Systems and Networking Support for Health Care and Assisted Living Environments, p. 4. ACM (2008)

40. Schouten, A.C., Boonstra, T.A., Nieuwenhuis, F., Campfens, S., van der Kooij, H.: A bilateral ankle manipulator to investigate human balance control. IEEE Trans. Neural Syst. Rehabil. Eng. 19(6), 660–669 (2011)

41. Khan, M.S.L., Lu, Z., Li, H., et al.: Head orientation modeling: Geometric head pose estimation using monocular camera. In: The 1st IEEE/IIAE International Conference on Intelligent Systems and Image Processing 2013, pp. 149–153 (2013)

42. Wang, G., Tao, Y., Yu, D., Cao, C., Chen, H., Yao, C.: Trainer: a motion-based interactive game for balance rehabilitation training. In: Proceedings of the Adjunct Publication of the 27th Annual ACM Symposium on User Interface Software and Technology, pp. 75–76. ACM (2014)

43. Wang, Y., Su, Y., Agrawal, G.: A novel approach for approximate aggregations over arrays. In: Proceedings of the 27th International Conference on Scientific and Statistical Database Management, p. 4. ACM (2015)

44. Wang, Y.-C., Huang, C.-K., Lee, W.-K., Hsu, Y.-P., Chen, L.-Y., Guo, H.-Y., Chang, Y.C., Wong, C.-L., Chiou, S.-C., Chang, J.-L., et al.: The convenient balance evaluation system. In: 2014 International Conference on Information Science, Electronics and Electrical Engineering (ISEEE), vol. 2, pp. 914–917. IEEE (2014)

45. Yang, J., Chen, B., Zhou, J., Lv, Z.: A low-power and portable biomedical device for respiratory monitoring with a stable power source. Sensors 15(8), 19618–19632 (2015)

46. Yang, J., Lin, Y., Gao, Z., Lv, Z., Wei, W., Song, H.: Quality index for stereoscopic images by separately evaluating adding and subtracting. PloS One 10(12), e0145800 (2015)

47. Yu, J., Skaff, S., Peng, L., Imai, F.: Leveraging knowledge-based inference for material classification. In: Proceedings of the 23rd Annual ACM Conference on Multimedia Conference, pp. 1243–1246. ACM (2015)

48. Yu, S., Ou, W., You, X., Mou, Y., Jiang, X., Tang, Y.: Single image rain streaks removal based on self-learning and structured sparse representation. In: 2015 IEEE China Summit and International Conference on Signal and Information Processing (ChinaSIP), pp. 215–219. IEEE (2015)

49. Yu, S., You, X., Zhao, K., Ou, W., Tang, Y.: Kernel normalized mixed-norm algorithm for system identification, pp. 1–6 (2015)

50. Zhang, S., Caragea, D., Ou, X.: An empirical study on using the national vulnerability database to predict software vulnerabilities. In: Hameurlain, A., Liddle, S.W., Schewe, K.-D., Zhou, X. (eds.) DEXA 2011. LNCS, vol. 6860, pp. 217–231. Springer, Heidelberg (2011). doi:10.1007/978-3-642-23088-2_15
51. Zhao, D., Zhang, Z., Zhou, X., Li, T., Wang, K., Kimpe, D., Carns, P., Ross, R., Raicu, I.: Fusionfs: toward supporting data-intensive scientific applications on extreme-scale high-performance computing systems. In: 2014 IEEE International Conference on Big Data (Big Data), pp. 61–70. IEEE (2014)

Model for Design of Serious Game for Rehabilitation in Children with Cochlear Implant

Sandra Cano[1(✉)], Victor Peñeñory[1], César Collazos[2],
Habib M. Fardoun[3], and Daniyal M. Alghazzawi[3]

[1] LIDIS Group, University of San Buenaventura, Cali, Colombia
Sandra.cano@gmail.com, vmpenenory@usbcali.edu.co
[2] IDIS Group, University of Cauca, Popayán, Colombia
ccollazo@unicauca.edu.co
[3] King Abdulaziz University, Jeddah, Saudi Arabia
{hfardoun,dghazzawi}@kau.edu.sa

Abstract. This paper presents a model based on Auditory-verbal therapy, which is carried out with deaf children who have benefited from a cochlear implant. These children must learn to acquire listening skills to develop their language. It is the speech therapist who helps the children during the rehabilitation process. A serious game could therefore help in the process of acquiring listening skills, wherein play activities are integrated but have a therapeutic effect. A model is presented here for the design of such a game. This model is based on an analysis of different types of game-therapy-player relationships, to identify the mechanics of the game and reliably build player profiles. All the inquiries are aimed at identifying different aspect between different types of game-therapy-player; to do this, 12 children from the Institute for Deaf and Blind Children, in Cali, Colombia participated, the children ranging from 7 to 11 years of age, all with a cochlear implant, where were analyzed a set of games for PC oriented toward speech therapy. The evaluations were made to identify different aspects like: users, game and pedagogical, in each action undertaken by the child on interact with the game. Finally it recreates a story through the character called Phonak who has become lost in a planet called Sounds and has to learn to listen in order to find his family. In turn, the game will help to develop not only speech and language skills but also cognitive ones. In this light, a serious game was put forward aimed at attracting the child's attention.

Keywords: Human computer interaction · Serious game · Auditory-verbal therapy · Children with cochlear implant

1 Introduction

The pronunciation of words by a non-hearing child is much more marked than that of children who hear. Early in the language acquisition process, children tend to repeat, imitating what they hear, words or entire sentences. This trend is more pronounced in children with cochlear implants [2]. Influential factors on the language problems of these children include the quality of their hearing with hearing aids before surgery, the age

© Springer International Publishing AG 2017
H.M. Fardoun et al. (Eds.): REHAB 2015, CCIS 665, pp. 94–105, 2017.
https://doi.org/10.1007/978-3-319-69694-2_9

they receive the implant, and the language level of the parents. Children given the implant earlier show a faster language development [2].

For children to learn, they must direct their attention and relate sounds to a word. That means they need to *listen*, not just hear; and to *look*, not just see [3]. Children, who are diagnosed at an early age with profound bilateral hearing loss are supported with hearing aids such as cochlear implants. Children who have been treated with cochlear implants can benefit significantly in AVT, but the therapy sessions are characterized by being highly repetitive, so that keeping patients motivated is difficult [1].

In the course of a speech therapy, the therapist usually makes use a variety of materials such as pictograms, papers, real objects, toys, and so on. It is often difficult for the therapist to create an appropriate environment for a particular therapy to achieve the hoped-for objective. Another problem for therapists concerns the preparation of a detailed report and delivery of a register of the therapy sessions carried out; all of which takes extra time. Thus, an environment of a game that includes the different activities that can be involved in their therapies, according to the needs of each child, could be of great help in supporting the rehabilitation process.

Today, digital games are considered as more than simply entertainment or leisure activities. Serious games are being used in different areas such as education, health, and in the military. Games that have a serious purpose beyond entertainment [5] are called *Serious Games* and defined as digital games with educational goals and that can act as an alternative in transmitting knowledge [15], which shows that the serious game integrates a relationship between two scenarios, a video-play-based scenario, where the aim is to have fun, and a pedagogical scenario, with an educational objective. In 2006, Michael and Chen [5] defined serious games as those used to educate, train and inform. Serious games is used to refer to applications developed through principles of technology and game design with a primary goal other than to entertain, having a link between the real and virtual world. For this reason, the design of serious games can offer healthy contributions in the area of rehabilitation, combining entertainment and education [4, 5], and these games can be integrated into the speech rehabilitation process.

Therapeutic games may be considered as serious games [20] that offer the twin scenarios of entertainment and therapy, and aim thereby to produce a particular desired effect that arises from a medical condition [18], without neglecting the aspect of motivation. The aim would thus be that the patient continue playing so as to complete tasks, over longer sessions, which are able to improve their medical condition. It is therefore necessary to identify aspects related to gameplay in therapy and patient motivation. The aim of this proposal is to build a model that will be of assistance in designing therapeutic games for children with cochlear implants.

Section 2 outlines the problem that therapists face when trying to adjust the appropriate settings for each therapy; Sect. 3 mentions the different contributions made for children with cochlear implants from voice therapy tools to games that interact with the voice to develop speech characteristics; Sect. 3 meanwhile gives a brief description of hearing rehabilitation for children with cochlear implants, which continues to be based on the AVT method; and in Sect. 4, the serious game prototype for AVT for children with Finally, the conclusions and future work to be carried out are described in Sect. 5.

2   Hearing Rehabilitation

Hearing rehabilitation in the patient begins the very moment the cochlear implant apparatus is switched on. It immediately begins to receive electrical stimuli that are perceived in the central nervous system. If the child already has auditory experience, the stimuli perceived are interpreted as auditory sensations. Otherwise, the stimuli are still perceived but provoke unknown sensations [14].

Hearing rehabilitation is known as the process by which children learn to use their hearing to the fullest. Therefore, the goal of rehabilitation is to help children learn to extract or draw information from the stimuli perceived via the cochlear implant. This process follows a number of steps responsible for developing various skills such as sound detection, sound identification, discrimination of phonemes, words and phrases, as well as understanding the oral message. This implies that rehabilitation involves AVT. With the support of educational materials, AVT stimulates the senses of the patient with the implant; hence the importance of having suitable material giving an optimal outcome in the patient as rehabilitation takes place.

3   Methodology

3.1   Model Proposed

The proposed model is a extension of the proposal put forward in [27] and also is based on the model proposed by [18], which establishes a relationship between *patient-game-therapy*. The objectives of the model are to involve the health expert in the process; identify a list of important aspects related to the game, patient and therapy; put in place design limitations using therapy-game-patient models, therapy-patient and patient-game relations. This model was proposed for adults with Alzheimer's. If it is used in children with hearing impairment it would be necessary to take other aspects into account, since the profile will be oriented toward children and there are different to those of adults.

At the same time, it was considered taking into account for the aspects of the game the MDA (Mechanics Dynamics and Aesthetics) model [19], designed by game designers. It has 3 levels of abstraction that can provide support for game design. Both of the above models were thus considered for adapting the proposed model according to the needs of a child with a cochlear implant.

Figure 1 shows the model that integrates the relationship between player-therapy, game-therapy, and player-game. The player-game relationship can be viewed as a cyclical process in which two active agents metaphorically listen, think and speak [17]. The game-therapy relationship on the other hand is related to how to integrate elements of motivation within the therapy without losing the effect of rehabilitation. Finally, the player-therapy relationship concerns itself with identifying the challenges and objectives that the player must complete in the course of the therapy.

Each established relationship considers aspects of game design in the context of rehabilitation. In the **player-game** relationship, information is captured about every action of the child on interacting with a set of existing games oriented toward speech

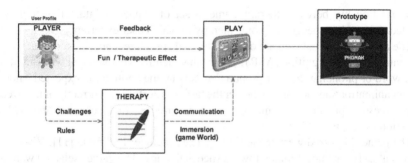

Fig. 1. Proposed model for design of a serious game in a therapy context.

therapy, in which different research techniques are applied such as direct observation, interviews, and tools to evaluate the child's experience with the game.

Meanwhile, the **therapy-game** relationship is concerned with the mechanics of the game, how to achieve an immersion of the child using the game, which challenges may be most appropriate, which communication strategies to use to achieve a result that is both fun and therapeutic. It is therefore important to consider that the story is related to the type of therapy to be undertaken, where different levels of progress in the therapy are to be considered as progress is made. In addition to the devices with which they will interact, it may be input or output material that enables the player to perceive the state of the game.

Finally, the **player-therapy** relationship comprises the different fun activities that the child undertakes that ought to produce a therapeutic effect on the child, since therapy as it stands has the goal of improving the condition of the patient. The speech therapist is thus involved as a medical expert in the design, communication, and strategies of the activities.

The results of applying the model to a group of children with cochlear implants from the institute for Deaf and Blind Children in the Cauca Valley are described below.

3.2 Participants

All the inquiries are aimed at building a profile of the player; to do this, 11 children from the Institute for Deaf and Blind Children, in Cali, Colombia participated, the children ranging from 7 to 11 years of age: (2) seven-year-old boys and old-girls; (4) eight-year-old boys; (2) nine-year-old boys; (1) nine-year-old boy; (2) eleven-year-old boys and old girls, who were in the academic years of transition, first and second grades of primary school.

3.3 Study Case

Applying the model to the case study, the player-game, therapy-game and player-therapy relationships were evaluated. To analyze the three relationships, different activities were carried out with the children to collect information about each of the relationships that can be established between child, therapy, and game. With the aim of seeking out aspects in the relationship between therapy-game, a set of games or interactive tools were selected, oriented to speech and voice therapy in which user experience was evaluated.

The applications analyzed are oriented toward speech technologies, so that they are automatic speech recognition (ASR) systems that identify a phoneme or word and verify if the word or phoneme the user pronounces is what the application expected, showing the user animations according to whether the task was performed correctly or incorrectly. To use these applications, a microphone is required as input channel and with the animation as output.

The games analyzed were made for PC. They include: Prelingua [11], Vivoso [13] and Vocaliza [6], games oriented toward speech therapy. The games selected were with support of the speech therapist, who is the person that taken the final decision, if the game can include into the therapy of child. Two assessment methods were applied, direct observation and cognitive walkthrough. Direct observation was used with the Vivoso game, an application that works on voice skills such as timbre, pitch, and intensity, where it has been identified that the type of technology used can affect the child's motivation. This could be seen when, after the children had been interacting with the PC it was decided to provide them with a Tablet to observe the children's behaviors and interests, and the effect produced was very positive compared to when they were carrying out their activities on the PC (Fig. 2). In addition, the children evaluated have an advanced level in therapy, since the activities for the training of listening skills are not a problem for them. This led to many of them performing the tasks more as a duty, and they were soon bored. Difficulties in using the mouse were also seen, so there was a heavy dependence on the evaluator in completing the activity.

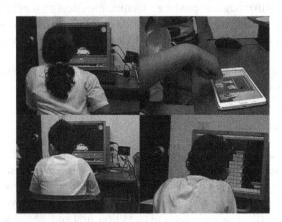

Fig. 2. Observing the different reactions between player-game.

Meanwhile, a user experience and usability assessment was made for the game entitled Pre-lingua [11], the main aspects of the voice that are worked in this game are detection, voice activity, intensity control, and breath control. Figure 3 shows the results obtained, where the test consists of a total of 50 questions, structured based on the QUIS [23], USE [24], GEQ [25] and UEQ [26] questionnaires, taking into account the effectiveness, efficiency, satisfaction, emotions and learning attributes. In the efficiency aspect, it can be seen that the results are almost identical, because most of the tasks performed with the children had not been adjusted to suit their learning level and were very easy for them. Facial expressions were thus not very significant as they completed the tasks without much effort. The aspect of learning also had an influence, with 48% of children achieving it without much difficulty. As a result, 47% was obtained for the emotions aspect, where the children showed greater degree of intensity in their emotions. This is because they found the game easy and they played it as though it were more of a mandatory activity, and not as though they were having fun.

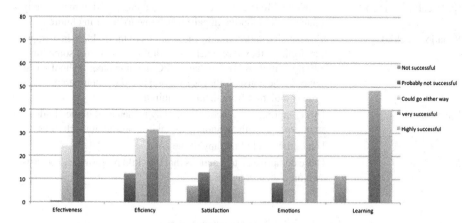

Fig. 3. Results of the evaluation of usability and user experience applied to the interactive tool called Pre-lingua.

An analysis of skills such as visual attention, visual perception, and memory was also carried out. These are fundamental for the development of their learning and for game design.

Using the data collection obtained from the various activities implemented with children aimed at evaluating the user experience, usability, cognitive processes and inclusion of information technology, different aspects were identified and analyzed different aspects in each action undertaken by the child on interact with the game and the player profile was built, shown in Table 1.

The aspects of the child that were analyzed were: behaviors, emotions, skills, interests and motivation, which help to structure the player profile for a specific context. In the activities carried out with the children, voice intensity control was evaluated. It was indicated to the child that they pronounce a consonant or vowel. According to the intensity registered, the visual element moved either forward or simply suspended in the air. A higher intensity moved the element forward. However, it was observed that when activities are repeated, the child displayed a rapid demotivation, so that performance in control of the game was reduced. Equally, the game only works on PC, so the child enjoyed greater motivation in interacting with a Tablet device included with the aim of identifying issues regarding the platform. As such, aspects of the therapy-game relationship were also identified (Table 2).

Table 1. Aspects of player profile.

Attributes	Description
Personal information	Involves important data that can offer support in defining the needs and learning level. These are: name, age, gender, and academic year
Skills/abilities	To find out skills that can be taken into account in establishing communication strategies
Disability (Physical/Cognitive)	Involves auditory physical disability as well as hearing loss (Mild, Moderate, Moderate-severe, Severe and Profound). It may equally relate to any cognitive impairment found to occur in children
Situation of child	It's related to understanding the situation of the children in therapy, the problems they face when the audiologist performs some fun activity with them. If they have a PC or some other technological device in the house. If they are accompanied by their parents, or if more stimulation from them is required
Emotions	This comprises the reactions that may be detected in the children on interacting with technology in their rehabilitation activities
Therapy Level	This is the level of therapy of the child
Motivation	These comprise certain actions that the child performs and persists with until their completion

Table 2. Therapy-game aspects

Attributes	Description
Learning curve	Refers to the level of experience of the child when interacting with Tablets as well as the level of therapy of the child according to their acquired skills. The system is responsible for controlling and setting learning with respect to the time spent and the resources used
Rules/challenges	These are subject to the goals to be achieved. They are the actions that the player can perform and actions that are not allowed
Reward	Positive scores obtained by carrying out an activity correctly
State of progress	Continuous feedback on the level reached as progress is made in the game
Gender	Elements common to both boys and girls, as in the virtual world
Dimensionality	Variables and laws that define aspects of the virtual world, such as: emotional, physical, temporal, among others

The relationship meanwhile between player-therapy (Table 3) basically comprises the different activities that the therapist should undertake with the child. These activities are repetitive since the aim is that the child should memorize the pronunciation and listening of different sounds. The children do not all have the same problem in relation to any given phoneme, so this type of rehabilitation cannot function cooperatively with other children. The activities carried out with children are so that they learn to identify sounds and pronounce them correctly, so that there are some important listening skills that the therapist must concentrate on in the early stages of the rehabilitation process so that the children acquire these. It is very important therefore to know in great detail what information the cochlear implant supplies to the child and what limitations in sound perception are involved. The therapy begins with detecting sounds, so such listening skills are worked on as auditory discrimination, auditory memory, auditory attention and foreground-background discrimination.

Table 3. Player-therapy aspects

Attributes	Description
Auditory perception	Implies recognizing, discriminating and interpreting auditory stimuli associated with previous experiences. It is the ability to give meaning to an auditory message
Auditory awareness	The ability to be aware that a sound is being made
Location of sound source	The ability to locate a sound or turn towards the source of a sound being produced
Auditory discrimination	The ability to differentiate between sounds
Foreground-background perception	The ability to direct perception to one part of the perceptual field, i.e. the foreground (sound) while treating the rest of the perceptive field as background
Auditory analysis and synthesis	The ability fully to break down auditory stimuli

Children with cochlear implants have a need to learn to listen, for this reason the tools presented had the objective of speech acquisition. In following the process of AVT, a serious game called "Training with Phonak" for Android Tablets is proposed. The game is based on the five stages of the rehabilitation process, these being detection, discrimination, identification, recognition, and comprehension. The aim is for these stages to become levels of therapy-learning, where children make progress by understanding and integrating the sounds through the entire process.

The "Training with Phonak" game recreates a story through the character called Phonak, who has become lost in a planet called Sounds and has to learn to listen in order to find his family (Fig. 4). To do this, he must travel to other planets and confront a variety of situations. As Phonak progresses during these levels, he will develop skills that will support him in acquiring the power of listening. He will have to travel through each planet and deal with situations that enable him to acquire skills related to detection, discrimination, identification, recognition, and listening comprehension. Each level has a set of activities that facilitates acquiring skills in listening and speaking.

For the construction of the scenario, it was considered taking into account the definition of serious game, which is defined with two scenarios, educational and recreational [14]. For this reason the game proposal is aimed at therapists in order that they might include the use of information technology in their rehabilitation, so that the patient does not quickly become demotivated. For the patient to be more motivated it is important to provide sufficient variability in the game and for the difficulty level to be adapted to the patient's behavioral observations.

Through the game it is hoped to improve perception and auditory discrimination, as well as the auditory memory of the child. In Fig. 4, the "detection" scenario is displayed. It is regarded as the first level of awareness or detection of the sound. For this reason, the child must listen to a series of items and in turn pronounce into the microphone to

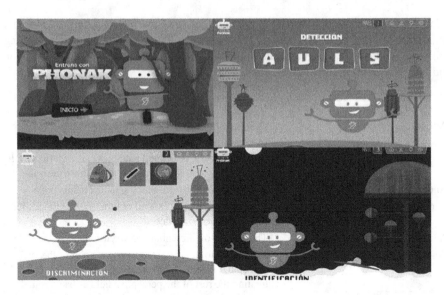

Fig. 4. Interface and levels of the "Training with Phonak" game for the Institute for Blind and Deaf Children from Cauca Valley.

allow interaction with the interface in a fun way. Following the learning method of Ling [3], in this first scenario the significant clues are represented for each frequency range, which using a set of phonemes the child must hear (detect) and then identify. The sounds that represent different frequency ranges are: A, U, L, S, SH, M, therefore the activity involves the child detecting the sound and associating it with the correct image the onomatopoeic sound represents. These tests should be performed from varying distances, usually with a male voice making the pronunciation of the sounds stronger or weaker, in order for the child to be able to listen at different distances. The sounds of Ling help in getting to know the hearing levels of the child.

In the discrimination scenario, a set of words is selected that are then played one by one, where children are asked to repeat what they hear. In the identification scenario, the P.I.P-S tests (word identification test using supra-segmentals) [22] are included. The word supgra-segmentals here refers to acoustic aspects such as accent, intonation and rhythm. The test consists of 12 stimuli with different patterns of stress and/or duration ordered randomly, these are: shoe, dolphin, flower, bottle cap, bread, paintbrush, button, pacifier, cheese, whistle and train, always accompanied by an image. It also includes the P.I.P-C tests (word identification test using Consonants) [21]. These words may vary according to age. The P.I.P-C test is used to find out if the child is able to make use of the information referring to the consonants. In the recognition stage come associated phrases. Understanding is related to sentences they are given to then carry out certain actions.

As a result, as the children progress though each stage of the therapy process, they will jump into each world. Each world in turn contains a set of tests that will be recorded as information for the audiologist.

4 Analysis and Discussion

Auditory-verbal therapy is a rehabilitation process that deaf children who have benefited from a cochlear implant require to undergo, since the aim of the therapy is for them to direct their attention and relate sounds to words. As such, they should listen, not simply hear; look, not just see. Most of these children have very specific problems particular to each, but if they acquire basic listening skills that allow them to develop speech, they will benefit significantly. As observed in the activities carried out with them geared to technology, they have shown that games can help during the rehabilitation process and could aid therapists as support material. The proposal is designed to be a mobile application, since that is where the best results were obtained for incorporating technology, in comparison with PCs, where it took a lot longer for them to manage the mouse.

In therapy, audiologists use a variety of materials, but they often need to create an environment that is suitable for a particular therapy, to achieve the desired outcome. Preparing a detailed report and making notes of all the therapy sessions conducted is a further problem facing therapists as all of this takes additional time. As a consequence, the player profile aspect has been set up with the aim of storing information about the player (the child) for each of the activities that they undertake, for which performance-measuring variables have been selected such as time, number of correct responses, number of incorrect responses, level, and so on, which will to some extent help identify aspects of therapy for each child and that will be of assistance to the audiologist.

5 Conclusions and Future Work

Games in therapy help increase motivation in the sessions. Therefore a serious game that involves two scenarios, educational and entertainment is able to support auditory-verbal therapy (AVT) for children with cochlear implants. In turn, the game will help to develop not only speech and language skills but also cognitive ones. In this light, a serious game was put forward aimed at attracting the child's attention, so that aspects of the game such as the progress acquired as advances are made in the game are considered, with the aim of producing in the child a sense of challenge, while allocating a score for each activity completed correctly.

The design of serious games is an area of research that is making use of design methodologies, interaction techniques, and technologies, among other tools, to help provide interactive applications in the area of rehabilitation. For this reason, as future work it is hoped to implement all the levels involved in the speech rehabilitation process and that these subsequently be evaluated with children, employing a design methodology for serious games aimed at children with hearing disabilities.

As future work it is hoped to apply the evaluation of the proposed game to a group of children with cochlear implants from the Institute of Blind and Deaf Children. It is also hoped to adapt variables that make it possible to adapt the therapy level and learning potential of the game.

References

1. Tan, C.T., Johnston, A., Ballard, K., Ferguson, S., Perera-Schulz, D.: sPeAK-MAN: towards popular gameplay for speech therapy. In: Proceedings of the 9th Australasian Conference on Interactive Entertainment: Matters of Life and Death (IE 2013). Article 28, 4 pages. ACM, New York (2013). http://doi.acm.org/10.1145/2513002.2513022
2. De Maggi, M.M.: Terapia Auditivo Verbal. Enseñar a escuchar para aprender hablar. Revista Electrónica de Audiología 2(3), 64–72 (2004)
3. Ling, D., Moheno, C.: El maravilloso sonido de la palabra. Programa Auditivo Verbal para niños, Editorial Trillas (2002)
4. Sawyer, B., Smith, P.: Serious games taxonomy. In: Serious Game Submmit, Game Developer Conference (2008)
5. Chen, S., Michael, D.: Serious Games: Games that Educate, Train and Inform. Thomson Course Technology, USA (2005)
6. Vaquero, C., Saz, O., Lleida, E., Rodríguez, W.R.: E-inclusion technologies for the speech handicapped. In: IEEE International Conference Acoustic, Speech and Signal Processing, pp. 4509–4512 (2008)
7. Speech Viewer. Product for speech language pathologists, teachers, and other professionals to use in modifying speech http://www.synapseadaptive.com/edmark/prod/sv3. visitado en junio del 2015
8. Wang, X., Jiang, F., Yang, D., Liu, M.: The application of cross recurrence plot in deaf linguistic training system. In: Bioinformatics and Biomedical Engineering, pp. 2020–2023 (2008)
9. Xu, W., Lifang, X., Dan, Y., Zhiyan, H.: Speech visualization based on robust selforganizing map (RSOM) for the hearing impaired. In: International Conference on Biomedical Engineering and Informatics, vol 2, pp. 506–509 (2008)
10. Sandra, C., Inés, Á.G., César, C., Jaime, A.M.: A proposal from visualization Human-Computer Interaction in the context of pronunciation information. J. VAEP-RITA 3(1), 14–20 (2015)
11. Rodríguez, W.R., Saz, O., Lleida, E.: A prelingual tool for the education of altered voices. Speech Commun. 54(5), 583–600 (2012)
12. Cano, S., Arteaga, J.M., Collazos, C.A., Bustos, V.A.: Model for analysis of Serious games for literacy in children from an User Experience approach. In: XVI International Conference on HCI, pp. 1–8 (2015)
13. Castillo, A.D.: Herramienta de software didáctica como soporte en la enseñanza del lenguaje oral para niños con deficiencia auditiva. En Primera ronda nacional de proyectos y realizaciones en tecnología biomédica. SENA Antioquia - Universidad de Antioquia - Univ. Pontificia Bolivariana - Univ. de San Buenaventura Medellín - Escuela de Ingeniería de Antioquia (2002)
14. Valenzuela, I.S.: Material didáctico para la terapia auditivo- verbal para niños con implante coclear del instituto "Audición, Voz y lenguaje AVYL". Tesis de licenciado en Diseño Gráfico. Universidad Vasco de Quiroga (2006)
15. Catalano, C.E., Luccini, A.M., Mortara, M.: Best practices for an effective design and evaluation of serious games. Int. J. Serious Games, 1–13 (2014)
16. Markopoulos, P., Read, J.C., MacFarlane, S., Hoysniemi, J.: Evaluating Children's Interactive Products: Principles and Practices for Interaction Designers. Morgan Kaufmann Publishers Inc., San Francisco (2008)
17. Crawford, C.: Chris Crawford on game design. New Riders Games, pp. 39–58 (2003)

18. Mader, S.: Le game design de jeux thérapeutiques Modèles et méthodes pour la conception du gameplay. Thèses de doctorat, École doctorale informatique, télécommunication et électronique, université de Paris
19. Hunicke, R., LeBlanc, M., Zubek, R.: MDA: A formal approach to game design and game research. In: Proceedings of the AAAI Workshop on Challenges in Game AI, vol. 4 (2004)
20. Alvarez, J., Djaouti, D.: Une Taxinomie des Serious Games dédiés au secteur de la santé. Revue de l'electricité et de l'electronique, société de l'electricité, de l'electronique et des technologies de l'information et de la communication (SEE), vol. 11, pp. 91–102 (2008)
21. Furmanski, H.M., Flandín, M.C., Howlin, M.I., Sterin, M.L., Yebra, S.: Prueba de identificación de palabras a través de consonantes. Edición del autor, Buenos Aíres, Argentina (1997)
22. Furmanski, H., Flandin, M., Howlin, M., Sterin, M., Yebra, S.: Test P.I.P. Prueba de identificación de palabras. Revista Fonoaudiológica. Asociación Argentina de Logopedia, Foniatría y Audiología, Tomo, vol. 43, no. 2, pp. 13–18 (1997)
23. Chin, J.P., Diehl, V.A., Norman, K.L.: Development of an instrument measuring user satisfaction of the human-computer interface. In: Proceedings of ACM CHI 1988 Conference on Human Factors in Computing Systems, pp. 213–218 (1988)
24. Lund, A.M.: Measuring usability with the USE questionnaire. STC Usability SIG Newsletter (2001)
25. Ijsselsteijn, W.A., de Kort, Y.A.W., Poels, K.: The game experience questionnaire: development of a self-report measure to assess the psychological impact of digital games (2008). Manuscript in preparation
26. Rauschenberger, M., Schrepp, M., Olschner, S., Thomaschewski, J., Cota, M.P.: Measurement of user experience. A Spanish Language version of the User Experience Questionnaire (UEQ). In: Rocha, A., Calvo-Manzano, J.A., Reis, L.P., Cota, M.P. (eds.) Sistemas y Tecnologías de Información- Actas de la 7a conferencia ibérica de Sistemas y Tecnologías de la Información (2012)
27. Cano, S., Peñeñory, V., Collazos, C.A., Fardoun, H.M., Alghazzawi, D.M.: Training with Phonak: serious game as support in auditory – verbal therapy for children with cochlear implants. In: Proceedings of the 3rd Workshop on ICTs for improving Patients Rehabilitation Research Techniques, pp. 22–25 (2015)

Hyperbaric Oxygen Chamber Users May Obtain Immersive Enjoyment by Virtual Reality Glasses

Zhihan Lv[✉]

FIVAN, Valencia, Spain
lvzhihan@gmail.com

Abstract. As for the users of hyperbaric oxygen therapy apartment, this paper put forward a newfangled immersing entertainment system. As for this system, it is a mixture of software and hardware, and this paper has depicted the scheme. And a HMD (i.e. virtual reality glasses shell), a water-repellent bag and a smart-phone compose the hardware. Besides, as for the software, it can transform the tridimensional images of the three-dimensional game into the smart-phone's screen at the same time. And in terms of the actual moving scene of the hospital hyperbaric oxygen treatment, people will talk about the option and comparison of the hardware. At last, it is likely to raise a rudimentary guideline to design this sort of system consequently.

Keywords: Virtual reality · HMD · Hyperbaric oxygen · Immersive

1 Introduction

The efficacy of hyperbaric oxygen therapy has been recorded in a lot of literature in clinical research community [9,33,34,38]. The limited space of the hyperbaric oxygen chamber has constrained the possibilities of activities. The most common activity that the users usually do in the hyperbaric oxygen chamber is sleeping, although the oxygen generation machine of the chamber is noisy which couldn't be ignored at all. Playing with smartphone or reading book also happens sometime, since they only need activities of upper arms. It's however still not comfortable to retain the postures of the upper arms and neck to play or read for long time. The physical discomforts may impair the psychological enjoyment. Overall, the spatial limitation constrains the physical activities inside the hyperbaric oxygen chamber. Our research plans to improve the user experience of hyperbaric oxygen therapy by novel virtual reality (VR) based interactive technologies, the imagination of the running scenario is shown as in Fig. 1.

Virtual reality (VR) environments are increasingly being used by neuroscientists [2] and psychotherapists [35] to simulate natural events and social interactions. VR technology has been proved to be able to stimuli for patients who has difficulty in imagining scenes and/or are too phobic to experience real situations since long time ago [31]. The 'Immersive' characteristic of VR technology

© Springer International Publishing AG 2017
H.M. Fardoun et al. (Eds.): REHAB 2015, CCIS 665, pp. 106–115, 2017.
https://doi.org/10.1007/978-3-319-69694-2_10

can substantially improve movement training for neurorehabilitation [1,5,15,29]. The report of the early research of utilizing VR to treat claustrophobia patient [3] has inspired our work, since the hyperbaric oxygen chamber is a typical sealed space. The underwater VR game for aquatic rehabilitation brings us some suggestions and tips [14] about the development of VR game on head mounted device (HMD) in unusual air environment (e.g. under water, in hyperbaric oxygen). Nonetheless, VR in clinical rehabilitation is still in infancy and need more exploration [32].

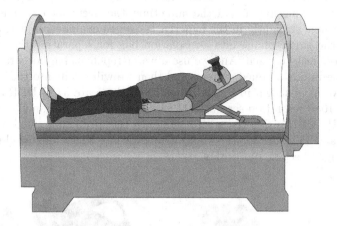

Fig. 1. The system running scenarios.

2   System

As for the users of hyperbaric oxygen therapy apartment, this paper put forward a newfangled immersing entertainment system. As for this system, it is a mixture of software and hardware, and this paper has depicted the scheme. And a HMD (i.e. virtual reality glasses shell), a water-repellent bag and a smart-phone compose the hardware. Besides, as for the software, it can transform the tridimensional images of the three-dimensional game into the smart-phone's screen at the same time. And in terms of the actual moving scene of the hospital hyperbaric oxygen treatment, people will talk about the option and comparison of the hardware. At last, it is likely to raise a rudimentary guideline to design this sort of system consequently. This paper is the extended version of our paper on Rehab2015 [18].

2.1   Hardware

As for the VR hardware, it has undergone the development of several generations. And at the same time, it has emerged some beneficial immersing circumstances, which includes the scope from inchoate surround-screen projection-based VR circumstance alleged CAVEE [6,7] to current human-computer-interface (HCI) like VR glasses. And for CAVE, it is unlikely for people to consider it into the hyperbaric oxygen chamber in that the cost is too high and it counts on the plane situation. Consequently, the best option to bring users who lie inside the hyperbaric oxygen chamber the three-dimensional immersing insight is VR glasses.

As for the scale and size of the hyperbaric oxygen chamber is 185 cm length, 90 cm diameter which cannot admit an adult. And the construction material of the chamber is plastic sheeting for reaching the goal of isolation. In addition, it owns 4 small windows on every side, which are shown in Fig. 3(C). For sake of preventing the explosion, and at the same time, the electronic device is not permitted to utilize straightly in the hyperbaric oxygen chamber, so it is necessary to seal up the smart-phone into an isolation bag for separating the cell phone to the high-density oxygen. And we use a water-repellent bag for wrapping the smart-phone in our planned system, and then we will set it into the HMD just like what we have shown in Fig. 2. In addition, there are 3 GB DDR3 memory, the 1920 * 1080 resolution screen, 441PPI, 95% NTSC color gamut, and Quad-Core 2.5 GHz CPU inside the smart-phone. In the mean time, it also supports Bluetooth and Wifi. As for the HMD configuration, those four productions as shown in Fig. 4 become our option.

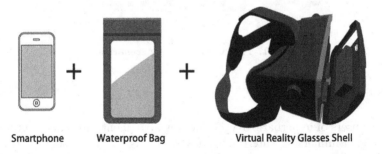

Smartphone   Waterproof Bag   Virtual Reality Glasses Shell

Fig. 2. Waterproof bag is employed to separate the phone to the high-density oxygen.

2.2 Software

In our system, the chosen smart-phone operates Android operating system. And it is possible to apply other smart-phone operating systems during future progress.

It is possible to enforce the three-dimensional utilizations on the screen of a smart-phone by using two sorts of software technologies just like what we have depicted as followed. Virtual Desktop. According to Fig. 3, the three-dimensional game GZ3DOOM, as the altered version of DOOM, is operating in three-dimensional mode. Besides, through a screen-real-time software, people can repeat the game window to the screen of a smart-phone. And Wifi has become the linkage between the PC and the smart-phone. And we utilized Trinus

VR [41] as the screen-real-time software containing an exe program operating on windows as server side and a .apk usage on the smart-phone as consumer side in our system. In addition, it is also likely to contact some other similar software by Google play, like Intugame VR [10]. What is worth mentioning is that TrinusVR owns pseudo three-dimensional function that is able to produce phony three-dimensional image through repeating the initial image voluntarily for every eye. Although the phony three-dimension practically brings users flat insight, there are also instruments which are able to transfer the switching from monoscopic of three-dimensional game to tridimensional side by side (SBS), such as Vireio [30] or TriDef 3D [39] and mobile phone app. It is likely for the three-dimensional game or VR scene usage operating on smart-phone to undergo worse performance of the system. And because the cumulative three-dimensional games on PC or other game devices in previous time are unable to operate on the smart-phone straightly or be ordinarily altered to be appropriate for the running system of the smart-phone (i.e. Android), the available usage resources are insufficient. In a word, through the following generation Cloud running system like Windows 10, a hopeful development trend of running system, it is possible for the user-defined mobile APP progressed for the smart-phone to promote better compatibility with the hardware. As for the current version of video game engines (i.e. Unity3D), the VR glasses SDK (i.e. Cardboard) have been offered to adjust to the present Unity3D APPs for fictitious actuality [11] that is a valid option accompanying with kind user interface for non-programmer.

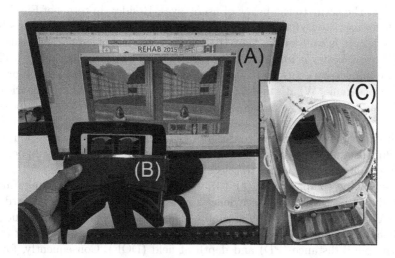

Fig. 3. The graphical content of screen (A) is duplicated to smartphone screen (B). (C) is the hyperbaric oxygen chamber located in our clinic.

2.3   Running Scenarios

In terms of Fig. 1, users (e.g. healthy people, patient, sportsman) can lie inside the hyperbaric oxygen chamber wearing the HMD and holding the remote controller. Furthermore, it is possible for users to play the three-dimensional game in three-dimensional mode or 2D game in pseudo three-dimensional mode that is able to show the image of game on the VR glasses. Furthermore, it is still likely to achieve the traditional need of reading E-books or getting into Internet basing on the VR glasses through pseudo 3D mode. And the motion of head and remote controller are contained in the input ways. Besides, the wheels around 3 axis controlled by gyroscope sensor of the smart-phone are just backed up by the head motion on VR glasses. Furthermore, the head motion is moved with the rotation of the avatar's horizon in the VR scene at the same time. That brings users the real-time immersing insight. In the mean time, people can use the remote controller to type in the displacement of the avatar and control the menu of the game shell.

3   Preliminary Comparison

According to Fig. 4, people will know the HMD which we have thought about and compared for the clinical necessity. And users are able to watch the anaglyph three-dimensional scene formed in the screen of a smart-phone from the VR glasses, namely are (a), (c), (d). However, (b) is alleged 'Lazy Glasses' whose lens reflect the scene to the below of users' eyes. Besides, in terms of Fig. 5, it is possible for users to lie flat and play the smart-phone rather than raise one's head or forearms. It is well-known that (b) is not a VR technology-oriented device, while it owns better conformity. Through wearing when one is raising neck or arms are unnecessary any more (b), it is likely for users to read a book or play smart-phone game. What's more, (b) is more handful and safe in hyperbaric oxygen chamber because it is a non-electronic device. Nevertheless, it is impossible for (b) to produce any three-dimensional images for immersing insight that is the critical term of VR. In a word, for users who do not actually want to undergo three-dimensional immersing process but still desire to read in the hyperbaric oxygen chamber, it is handful to select (b).

After having compared (a), (c), (d), we have known that the 3 configurations are produced by hard plastic, ethylene-vinyl acetate (EVA), and cardboard severally. And to block lightly, the assembly-to-appearance part of (a) is produced by soft holster filling of sponge. Thus, it is light. Besides, it is possible for (a) to alter the pupil distance (PD) and depth of field (DOF). Consequently, for the users who have diverse myopia degree and PD, (a) is suitable. And for users who are different in physical features, (c) and (d) have insufficient accommodative functions in that both are no matter how in folding structures the transportability of which causes convenience for allocation and transportation. In terms of our actual clinical need, it is more suitable for various patients to choose the characteristics of (b). At the same time, it is almost same for the price level of the 4 devices chosen by us. Thus, the incentive of the device option in future actual use will not be influenced by the cost problem.

And the dizziness is the general shortcoming of the HMDs which is largely induced by the vision delay that causes the imbalance of cochlear and vestibular. Furthermore, in terms of our case, lying posture does not cause more dizziness than other postures like sitting and standing. Therefore, we have a belief that as for hyperbaric oxygen chamber users, the VR glasses will produce immersing amusement provided that it is able to produce enjoyment to ordinary players.

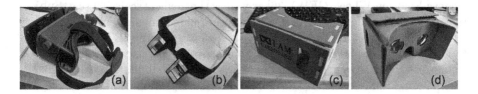

Fig. 4. The HMD that we have considered and compared for the clinical need.

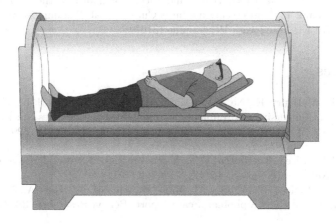

Fig. 5. The user is experiencing 'Lazy Glasses' and playing with mobile phone.

4 Designing Guideline

1. The water proof bag is necessary for isolation from hyperbaric oxygen.
2. It's significant to choose a comfortable HMD shell.
3. The smartphone programming doesn't have to be done as long as a PC or laptop is nearby as a server.
4. An additional remote controller is needed for menu manipulation.
5. Dizziness is not enhanced by hyperbaric oxygen chamber.
6. 'Lazy Glasses' is a non-electrical choice for users who hope to read 2D content.

5 Conclusion

In this paper, we proposed a hybrid system for improving the user experience in the hyperbaric oxygen chamber. By this system, users can enjoy 3D stereoscopic games wearing virtual reality glasses and immersive perception, as well as read E-books or play the 2D games. Several HMDs have been tested and compared by us. All the technical issues have been solved, the new challenges are the customized 3D games or software used for this case. The efficacy of this system will be evaluated in future research by subjective measurement such as Geneva Emotion Wheel (GEW) [36] as well as the medical scales [3] (e.g. Subjective units of discomfort scale (SUDS), Problem-related impairment questionnaire (PRIQ), Self-efficacy towards the target behavior measure (SETBM), The attitude towards CTS measure (TAM)). Some novel technology will also be used to improve this research, e.g., Sensors [42], Virtual Rehabilitation [20,21,26,27], HCI [22–25,37], Multimedia [4,17,28,43], Database [40,44], Big Data [19,45,46], Network [12,13,16], Optimization Algorithm [8].

Acknowledgment. The authors would like to thank Pablo Gagliardo and Sonia Blasco for practical clinical suggestions and fruitful discussion about the technical possibility, and thank Dr. Javier Chirivella and Vicente Penades for the help at FIVAN. The authors thank to LanPercept, a Marie Curie Initial Training Network funded through the 7th EU Framework Programme (316748).

References

1. Bajcsy, P., McHenry, K., Na, H.-J., Malik, R., Spencer, A., Lee, S.-K., Kooper, R., Frogley, M.: Immersive environments for rehabilitation activities. In: Proceedings of the 17th ACM International Conference on Multimedia, pp. 829–832. ACM (2009)
2. Bohil, C.J., Alicea, B., Biocca, F.A.: Virtual reality in neuroscience research and therapy. Nat. Rev. Neurosci. **12**(12), 752–762 (2011)
3. Botella, C., Baños, R., Perpina, C., Villa, H., Alcaniz, M., Rey, A.: Virtual reality treatment of claustrophobia: a case report. Behav. Res. Ther. **36**(2), 239–246 (1998)
4. Chen, Z., Huang, W., Lv, Z.: Towards a face recognition method based on uncorrelated discriminant sparse preserving projection. Multimed. Tools Appl. pp. 1–15 (2015)
5. Connelly, L., Jia, Y., Toro, M.L., Stoykov, M.E., Kenyon, R.V., Kamper, D.G.: A pneumatic glove and immersive virtual reality environment for hand rehabilitative training after stroke. IEEE Trans. Neural Syst. Rehab. Eng. **18**(5), 551–559 (2010)
6. Cruz-Neira, C., Sandin, D.J., DeFanti, T.A.: Surround-screen projection-based virtual reality: the design and implementation of the cave. In: Proceedings of the 20th Annual Conference on Computer Graphics and Interactive Techniques, SIGGRAPH 1993, pp. 135–142. ACM, New York (1993)
7. Cruz-Neira, C., Sandin, D.J., DeFanti, T.A., Kenyon, R.V., Hart, J.C.: The cave: audio visual experience automatic virtual environment. Commun. ACM **35**(6), 64–72 (1992)

8. Dang, S., Ju, J., Matthews, D., Feng, X., Zuo, C.: Efficient solar power heating system based on lenticular condensation. In: 2014 International Conference on Information Science, Electronics and Electrical Engineering (ISEEE), vol. 2, pp. 736–739, April 2014
9. Davis, J.C., Hunt, T.: Hyperbaric oxygen therapy. J. Intensive Care Med. **4**(2), 55–57 (1989)
10. Georgi, G., Krasimir, N.: Intugame VR. http://intugame.com
11. Google: Cardboard SDK for unity. https://developers.google.com/cardboard/unity/
12. Jiang, D., Xu, Z., Lv, Z.: A multicast delivery approach with minimum energy consumption for wireless multi-hop networks. Telecommun. Syst. pp. 1–12 (2015)
13. Jiang, D., Ying, X., Han, Y., Lv, Z.: Collaborative multi-hop routing in cognitive wireless networks. Wirel. Pers. Commun. pp. 1–23 (2015)
14. John, Q.: Shark punch: a virtual reality game for aquatic rehabilitation. In: Virtual Reality (VR), pp. 265–266. IEEE (2015)
15. Kizony, R., Katz, N., et al.: Adapting an immersive virtual reality system for rehabilitation. J. Vis. Comput. Animat. **14**(5), 261–268 (2003)
16. Li, T., Zhou, X., Brandstatter, K., Zhao, D., Wang, K., Rajendran, A., Zhang, Z., Raicu, I.: ZHT: a light-weight reliable persistent dynamic scalable zero-hop distributed hash table. In: IEEE 27th International Symposium on Parallel & Distributed Processing (IPDPS), pp. 775–787. IEEE (2013)
17. Liu, Y., Yang, J., Meng, Q., Lv, Z., Song, Z., Gao, Z.: Stereoscopic image quality assessment method based on binocular combination saliency model. Signal Process. **125**, 237–248 (2016)
18. Lv, Z.: Bringing immersive enjoyment to hyperbaric oxygen chamber users using virtual reality glasses. In: Proceedings of the 3rd 2015 Workshop on ICTs for Improving Patients Rehabilitation Research Techniques, pp. 156–159. ACM (2015)
19. Lv, Z., Chirivella, J., Gagliardo, P.: Bigdata oriented multimedia mobile health applications. J. Med. Syst. **40**(5), 1–10 (2016)
20. Lv, Z., Esteve, C., Chirivella, J., Gagliardo, P.: Clinical feedback and technology selection of game based dysphonic rehabilitation tool. In: 9th International Conference on Pervasive Computing Technologies for Healthcare (PervasiveHealth2015). IEEE (2015)
21. Lv, Z., Esteve, C., Chirivella, J., Gagliardo, P.: A game based assistive tool for rehabilitation of dysphonic patients. In: 2015 3rd IEEE VR International Workshop on Virtual and Augmented Assistive Technology (VAAT), pp. 9–14, March 2015
22. Lv, Z., Feng, L., Li, H., Feng, S.: Hand-free motion interaction on Google glass. In: SIGGRAPH Asia 2014 Mobile Graphics and Interactive Applications. ACM (2014)
23. Lv, Z., Feng, S., Feng, L., Li, H.: Extending touch-less interaction on vision based wearable device. In: Virtual Reality (VR), pp. 231–232. IEEE, March 2015
24. Lv, Z., Feng, S., Khan, M.S.L., Ur Réhman, S., Li, H.: Foot motion sensing: augmented game interface based on foot interaction for smartphone. In: CHI 2014 Extended Abstracts on Human Factors in Computing Systems, pp. 293–296. ACM (2014)
25. Lv, Z., Halawani, A., Feng, S., Ur Réhman, S., Li, H.: Touch-less interactive augmented reality game on vision-based wearable device. Pers. Ubiquitous Comput. **19**(3–4), 551–567 (2015)

26. Lv, Z., Penades, V., Blasco, S., Chirivella, J., Gagliardo, P.: Comparing Kinect2 based balance measurement software to Wii balance board. In: Proceedings of the 3rd 2015 Workshop on ICTs for Improving Patients Rehabilitation Research Techniques, pp. 50–53. ACM (2015)

27. Lv, Z., Penades, V., Blasco, S., Chirivella, J., Gagliardo, P.: Intuitive evaluation of Kinect2 based balance measurement software. In: Proceedings of the 3rd 2015 Workshop on ICTs for Improving Patients Rehabilitation Research Techniques, pp. 62–65. ACM (2015)

28. Lv, Z., Tek, A., Da Silva, F., Empereur-Mot, C., Chavent, M., Baaden, M.: Game on, science-how video game technology may help biologists tackle visualization challenges. PLoS ONE 8(3), e57990 (2013)

29. Munih, M., Riener, R., Colombo, G., Lünenburger, L., Müller, F., Slater, M., Mihelj, M.: Mimics: multimodal immersive motion rehabilitation of upper and lower extremities by exploiting biocooperation principles. In: IEEE International Conference on Rehabilitation Robotics. ICORR 2009, pp. 127–132. IEEE (2009)

30. Neil, S.: Vireio. http://www.mtbs3d.com/new-vireio-site

31. North, M.M., North, S.M., Coble, J.R.: virtual reality therapy: an effective treatment for psychological disorders. Stud. Health Technol. Inform. 44, 59–70 (1997)

32. Ottosson, S.: Virtual reality in the product development process. J. Eng. Des. 13(2), 159–172 (2002)

33. Grim, P.S., Gottlieb, L.J., Boddie, A., Batson, E.: Hyperbaric oxygen therapy. JAMA 263(16), 2216–2220 (1990)

34. Ingle, R.: Hyperbaric oxygen therapy. JAMA 264(14), 1811 (1990)

35. Riva, G.: Virtual reality in psychotherapy: review. Cyberpsychology Behav. 8(3), 220–230 (2005)

36. Scherer, K.R.: What are emotions? And how can they be measured? Soc. Sci. Inf. 44(4), 695–729 (2005)

37. Khan, M.S.L., Lu, Z., Li, H., et al.: Head orientation modeling: geometric head pose estimation using monocular camera. In: The 1st IEEE/IIAE International Conference on Intelligent Systems and Image Processing, pp. 149–153 (2013)

38. Tibbles, P.M., Edelsberg, J.S.: Hyperbaric-oxygen therapy. New Engl. J. Med. 334(25), 1642–1648 (1996). PMID: 8628361

39. TriDef: TriDef 3D. https://www.tridef.com

40. Wang, Y., Su, Y., Agrawal, G.: A novel approach for approximate aggregations over arrays. In: Proceedings of the 27th International Conference on Scientific and Statistical Database Management, p. 4. ACM (2015)

41. Xavier, S.: Trinus VR. http://trinusvr.com

42. Yang, J., Chen, B., Zhou, J., Lv, Z.: A low-power and portable biomedical device for respiratory monitoring with a stable power source. Sensors 15(8), 19618–19632 (2015)

43. Yang, J., Lin, Y., Gao, Z., Lv, Z., Wei, W., Song, H.: Quality index for stereoscopic images by separately evaluating adding and subtracting. PLoS ONE 10(12), e0145800 (2015)

44. Zhang, S., Caragea, D., Ou, X.: An empirical study on using the national vulnerability database to predict software vulnerabilities. In: Hameurlain, A., Liddle, S.W., Schewe, K.-D., Zhou, X. (eds.) DEXA 2011. LNCS, vol. 6860, pp. 217–231. Springer, Heidelberg (2011). doi:10.1007/978-3-642-23088-2_15

45. Zhang, S., Zhang, X., Ou, X.: After we knew it: empirical study and modeling of cost-effectiveness of exploiting prevalent known vulnerabilities across iaas cloud. In: Proceedings of the 9th ACM symposium on Information, Computer and Communications Security, pp. 317–328. ACM (2014)
46. Zhao, D., Zhang, Z., Zhou, X., Li, T., Wang, K., Kimpe, D., Carns, P., Ross, R., Raicu, I.: FusionFS: toward supporting data-intensive scientific applications on extreme-scale high-performance computing systems. In: IEEE International Conference on Big Data (Big Data), pp. 61–70. IEEE (2014)

Amblyopia Rehabilitation by Games for Low-Cost Virtual Reality Visors

Silvia Bonfanti and Angelo Gargantini[✉]

Università degli Studi di Bergamo, Bergamo, Italy
{silvia.bonfanti,angelo.gargantini}@unibg.it
http://3d4amb.unibg.it

Abstract. Amblyopia is the partial or complete loss of vision in one eye (called *lazy eye*). It can be prevented by adequate treatment during the first years of young age. However, the classical therapy of eye patching suffers from a low compliance that can harm the treatment. To increase compliance, we have devised a system based on the combined use of low cost virtual reality visors, like the Google Cardboard, and ad hoc developed games for smartphones. Our system exploits the visor in order to send to the lazy eye an enhanced version of the gaming image while it sends to the normal eye a weakened version of the same image. In this way, the lazy eye must work more than the normal eye. We present here the principles, some issues we encountered, the integration of the games with a service that collects the data, and two games, namely a car racing and a tetris game.

Keywords: Amblyopia · Cardboard · Virtual reality visor · Rehabilitation · Android · Mobile games

1 Introduction

Amblyopia, otherwise known as 'lazy eye', is reduced visual acuity that results in poor or indistinct vision in one eye that is otherwise physically normal. It may exist even in the absence of any detectable organic disease. Amblyopia is generally associated with a squint or unequal lenses in the prescription spectacles. This low vision is not correctable (or only partially) by glasses or contact lenses. Amblyopia is caused by media opacity, strabismus, anisometropia, and significant refractive errors, such as high astigmatism, hyperopia, or myopia. This condition affects 2–3% of the population, which equates to conservatively around 10 million people under the age of 8 years worldwide [13]. If amblyopia is not diagnosed and treated in the first years of life, the lazy eye becomes weaker and the normal eye becomes dominant. The traditional way to treat amblyopia is carried out wearing a patch over the normal eye for several hours a day, through a treatment period of several months. This treatment has some drawbacks: it is unpopular, not well accepted by the young patients, and sometimes can disrupt the residual fusion between the eyes.

© Springer International Publishing AG 2017
H.M. Fardoun et al. (Eds.): REHAB 2015, CCIS 665, pp. 116–125, 2017.
https://doi.org/10.1007/978-3-319-69694-2_11

Our group has been involved in the use of computer technologies for the treatment of amblyopia for several years. The project 3D4AMB[1] exploits the stereoscopic 3D technology, that through glasses with LCD active shutters permits to show different images to the amblyopic eye and the normal eye. We developed some software both for amblyopia diagnosis [5] and treatment that uses this kind of 3D technology [11]. A form of treatment we have proposed, consists in watching video clips with 3D glasses that realize a virtual visual rebalancing [4]. Note that the classic use of a 3D system (like 3D glasses or Virtual Reality visors like the Oculus Rift) is to provide different images to the two eyes of the same scene with viewing angles slightly out of phase, that correspond to the different points of view of left and right eye. This vision produces an illusion of depth of the scene and is the heart of virtual reality. The primary principle of the system is that the images shown to the two eyes are different but related.

In this project, we exploit 3D systems in order to send two different images to the two eye not in order to provide an illusion of depth but to stimulate the lazy eye to exercise more than the normal eye. In this work we plan to advance w.r.t. the existing treatments by using a much cheaper virtual reality device (already used for screening amblyopia [2]) and by increasing the level of activity required from the patients. Indeed, while patching and vision rebalancing are classified as passive method, other treatments which require some activity on the part of the patients are classified as *active*. Active methods are intended to enhance treatment of amblyopia in a number of ways, including increased compliance and attention during the treatment periods (due to activities that are interesting for the patient) and the use of stimuli designed to activate and to encourage connectivity between certain cortical cell types. A good survey and assessment about active treatments and their efficiency can be found in [9].

The active treatment proposed in this paper consists in playing with interactive games or exercises, which will stream binocular images. In this settings, the child plays with a special video game which will exploit the binocular vision to send to the lazy eye all the details while the normal eye will see only a part of the game scene. To successfully complete the game or the exercise the patient must use the information shown to the lazy eye (and possibly fuse it with the information shown to the normal eye). In this way, the amblyopic eye is more stimulated and the fusion encouraged. The game application must continuously monitor the success rate of the game in order to adjust the difficulty based on the real capability of the player. It is well known that video games can be very useful for visual rehabilitation [1]. Classical examples of games found in literature, include PAC-MAN and simple car racing games [12]. This work extends the work presented in [6] by introducing a tetris game (similarly to [10]) besides a simple car racing game.

In this paper, first in Sect. 2, we introduce low cost virtual visors like the Google Cardboards and explain how they work. Then, in Sect. 3, we explain how gaming with this devices can be exploited for our goals. Sections 4 and 5 introduce our two mobile applications that realize the video game for amblyopia treatment.

---

[1] http://3d4amb.unibg.it/.

2   Low-Cost Virtual-Reality Visors

The Google Cardboard platform pioneered the use of low-cost devices for virtual reality (VR). These devises are made by inexpensive material and require the combined use of a smartphone in order to work. The Google Cardboard has been developed by Google and it was created by David Coz and Damien Henry, Google engineers at the Google Cultural Institute in Paris, in their 20% "Innovation Time Off" [8], and introduced at the Google I/O 2014 developers conference for Android devices. It is intended as a low-cost system to encourage interest and development in VR and VR applications [3].

It consists of a fold-out cardboard with two lenses where the user must insert the smartphone (see Fig. 1). While the original device is made by actual cardboard, nowadays plastic devices can be easily found for a price in the order of 30 dollars.

The working principle is simple: the user looks inside in order to see the images displayed by the phone. It permits a stereo vision by sending two different images to the two eyes. It works with different smartphones and can be easily adapted to be used by children. The system proposed in this paper also works with other types of VR viewers (e.g., Samsung Gear VR).

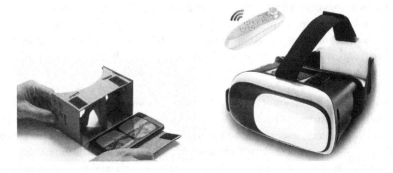

Fig. 1. The original Google Cardboard VR visor and a plastic variant

It is not an experience as the strap-on Oculus Rift headset, which requires a computer (and is still in development), or Samsung Gear VR, which costs $200 and only works with the Galaxy Note 4. But it is an easy way to get a feel for what is possible with modern virtual reality, and beyond the low cost of the headset, most of the available apps are free.

3   Low-Cost VR Games for Amblyopia Rehabilitation

In this section we explain how we can exploit low cost VR devices presented in the previous section for our goals. We will discuss the principles, the challenges, and how this system has been integrated in a service able to track the patient exercises and progress.

3.1   Using Low-Cost VR for Amblyopia Rehabilitation

Low-cost VR devices can show 3D images by displaying on the phone two different images in the two parts of the screen. This principle can be used in practice also for the treatment of amblyopia by sending two different images to the two eyes: the game app will show the most interesting part of the frame of the clip or game to the amblyopic eye, while we will show the least interesting part to the not amblyopic eye (or good). The principle, in case of use of the Google Cardboard is depicted in Fig. 2. Since the patients are young children, we decided to implement the diagnosis and treatment modules in a form of simple videogames, in order to make the treatment fun and not boring. The final aim of the project is to give the patients a complete system for the treatment that can be used at home. In fact, a smartphone and an inexpensive Google Cardboard are enough to run the software presented in this paper.

Our project follows the recent trend of using inexpensive technologies for amblyopia rehabilitation. Other approaches are based on the use of anaglyph glasses [7,14]. The main advantages of our approach is that the colour of the images is not change, providing in this way a better experience.

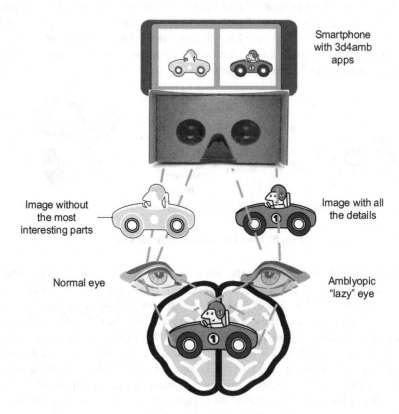

Fig. 2. 3D4Amb system with Google Cardboard

3.2   Interaction with Games Using Google Cardboard

User interaction is not easy because the smartphone is inside the Google Card-board and the user cannot tap on the screen. We have run up against this problem during the Stereoacuity Test development [2]. To avoid this limitation we suggest and now support several solutions:

- Stereo headset buttons (Fig. 3a and b)
- Bluetooth remote controller (Fig. 3c)
- Speech-controller

The simplest solution is to use standard *stereo headset*. Stereo headset usable for our applications must contains three buttons, i.e. plus button (+), minus button (−) and answer button. These buttons can be used to perform different actions in the games. The disadvantage with stereo headset is that the buttons are too small and too close, this can cause wrong push during the games. Wired earphones (Fig. 3a) has also the problem that the wires can obstacle the use of the VR device. To avoid this problem, bluetooth wireless earphones can be used instead since they provide a controller (Fig. 3b) for the earphones that can be used to control our applications.

A more specialized version is a *bluetooth remote controller* that is a special purpose device as presented in Fig. 3c. It has more than three buttons and it allows to perform more actions. The market offers different type of bluetooth remote controller, complex and easier, and this allows the developer to choose the one more suitable for the application.

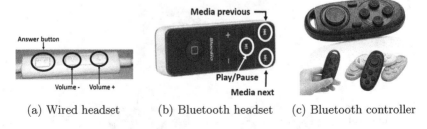

(a) Wired headset   (b) Bluetooth headset   (c) Bluetooth controller

Fig. 3. User interaction with games

Another possibility is to use the voice to control the games. This software *speech-controller* allows the user to interact with the application using the voice. There are some available libraries that given sounds translate them into words and the developer can take these words to perform some actions. We have tested two libraries: Android speech recognizer and CMUSphinx. The former works well, but has a bug: after few seconds of silent the speech recognizer crashes and it is not able to continue to take commands. The latter is developed for research projects and has more modules to allows the development of different functionalities. We have tried the second approach with our applications, but we met the following problems: 1. the system does not recognise words if background noise is present 2. the system is slow in processing sounds.

3.3   Traceability of User Improvements

During the therapy execution the user is interested in keeping track of his improvement. We have developed a web service that collects games results. Our games interact with this service in order to send data. Before starting the results saving process, the user has to make the registration using the "SIGN UP" button (Fig. 4a). Some information are required to complete the registration, i.e., email, password, name, surname and age. The email and the password, chosen during the registration, are used to LOGIN before the start of the game. At the end of the game the data are sent to the server and the user can ask to receive an email with a summary of the performance to understand if he is getting better. It is available the possibility to play without registration, but this does not allow to trace improvements.

Sometimes could happen that the doctors want to follow the patient improvement during some test sessions in their office. The game applications provide a doctor interface (Fig. 4b) to manage the patients results. The doctor registers using email and password. After the LOGIN, he can choose the patient for treatment session, add patients and check their improvements.

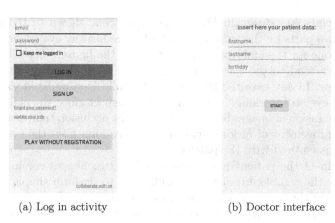

(a) Log in activity   (b) Doctor interface

Fig. 4. Interaction with games

4   Car Racing Mobile Application for Amblyopia Treatment

The principle of using 3D for penalization of the normal eye in amblyopic children, as explained before, has been applied in the game development for the treatment of amblyopia. The game is called *Car Racing Cardboard (CRC)* which works for the Google Cardboard and it is freely available on the Google play store[2]. The goal of this game is to avoid cars coming from the opposite side. The difficult of the game will increase when the user passes to next levels.

---

[2] https://play.google.com/store/apps/details?id=it.unibg.p3d4amb.
carracingcarboard.

Required Hardware. The CRC application has been developed for Android system. The basic hardware needed to use the game is: Android Smartphone (with the CRC application installed), Google Cardboard, or any other 3D VR glasses and earphone with controller (+, − and confirm) to play with the game.

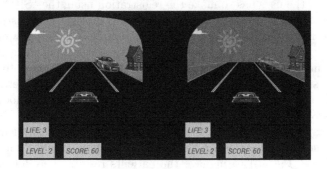

Fig. 5. A simple game scene of CRC

Game Principle. As shown in Fig. 5, the game scene shown to the patient is divided in two parts by the application, one for the healthy eye (right eye in the figure) and one for the amblyopic eye (left eye in the figure). The CRC decides which images send to the eyes depending on the type of treatment suggested by the doctor. In any case the lazy eye of the child is stimulated to work and the healthy eye still working. This is a positive aspect since the child does not interrupt the fusion of images between the eyes (the occlusion treatment does not help the improvement of fusion between images coming from the eyes, because the healthy is covered with the patch).

The brain of the patient has to combine the two images coming from the eyes to view the complete frame successfully and to perform simple operations like identifying the incoming cars and move the main car. There is a significant number of common elements between left and right images in order to make sure that the patient can merge them. The final frame is not a 3D-dimensional representation since the objective is not to stimulate the stereo vision of the patient (at least initially), but to make the eyes working together in the same way.

Game Description. Before the beginning of game, the application allows the user to choose the lazy eye (left or right), in order to decide between two different views (penalize the right or left eye). The goal of the game consists in getting the highest score possible. The gamer moves the main car (in the bottom of the view) in order to avoid obstacles (i.e. incoming cars in the opposite direction), and if it does not hit any obstacle, the score increases. When the child avoids a predetermine number of cars, the level increases. When the level rises, the speed and the number of obstacles increase so as to make the game more difficult. However, the most important aspect is given by the dynamic penalization of the scene shown to the healthy eye. In fact, when the level rises, the application increases the transparency of the panorama and the obstacles displayed for the not amblyopic eye, in order to train the lazy eye. The game ends after 3 collisions (after 3 lives lost). The gamer uses earphone to play. "+" and "−" buttons are used to choose the lazy eye at the beginning of the game and to move the main car in order to avoid obstacles. Instead, confirm button is used to start the game or restart it after the end. If the user is logged into the application, at the end of each game session the data are saved to track the improvement.

5   Tetris for Amblyopia Treatment

As the CRC game, Tetris has been developed for the treatment of amblyopia (Fig. 6). The goal of the game is like the original. The screen is split into two parts, one for the left eye and one for the right eye. The blocks get down and the user has to move them in the correct position in order to delete the lower rows. The blocks are not shown with the same definition to both eye, for the healthy eye they are degraded. In this way the amblyopic eye has to work harder to allow the correct recognition of blocks position. The brain combines the images coming from the eyes to rebuild the complete image. At the beginning the game is easier because the image sent to the healthy eye is slightly degraded. When the user deletes lower rows, the difficulty increases and the image sent to the healthy eye is more degraded. At the end of the game, if the user has logged in, the score is saved and is sent to the server. The gamer uses earphone to play. "+" button moves the blocks on the left, "−" button moves the blocks on the right and confirmed button rotates the blocks. As for the CRC, the user is able to follow his improvement during the treatment.

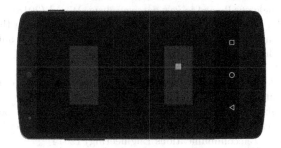

Fig. 6. A tetris cardboard game

6   Conclusion and Future Work

The aim of the two applications shown in previous sections is the treatment of amblyopia (or lazy eye). They require the use of inexpensive devices: a visor and stereo headset. By using the applications, people with lazy eye can improve their vision in the lazy eye. The policy for the treatment of amblyopia proposed by

3D4Amb, also tries to avoid the classical risks of the patch therapy (poor conformance and fusion disruption) and allows a interactive and supervised healing. However, at least initially, this therapy can be performed alongside with the classical occlusion. Although there are not clinical results available at the moment to support the effectiveness of the application, a series of experiments with children are currently carried on at the local hospital in order to check the validity and viability of the proposed approach. At the moment, the system for registration provides the possibility to save the results and check them by email. Feature development will be done in order to offer this service on a web server. We are planning to develop a platform where user can register. Once he is registered can use the same credentials for all games. A web application will be available to consult the results reached in different games during the treatment. A collaboration with some medical centers is going to start with the target to collect data from patients. It is also interesting to analyze how long the child needs to play before achieve some clinical improvement and how this method could replace or help current therapies.

Acknowledgments. Authors would like to thank Fabio Terzi and Matteo Zambelli for their work on this project.

References

1. Achtman, R., Green, C., Bavelier, D.: Video games as a tool to train visual skills. Restor. Neurol. Neurosci. **26**(4–5), 435–446 (2008)
2. Bonfanti, S., Gargantini, A., Vitali, A.: A mobile application for the stereoacuity test. In: Duffy, V.G. (ed.) DHM 2015. LNCS, vol. 9185, pp. 315–326. Springer, Cham (2015). doi:10.1007/978-3-319-21070-4_32
3. David, P.: Google cardboard is vr's gateway drug. Wired (2015)
4. Gargantini, A., Bana, M., Fabiani, F.: Using 3D for rebalancing the visual system of amblyopic children. In: 2011 International Conference on Virtual Rehabilitation (ICVR), Zurich, pp. 1–7, June 2011
5. Gargantini, A., Facoetti, G., Vitali, A.: A random dot stereo acuity test based on 3D technology. In: Proceedings of the 8th International Conference on Pervasive Computing Technologies for Healthcare - 2nd Patient Rehabilitation Research Techniques Workshop, PervasiveHealth 2014, pp. 358–361, ICST, Brussels, Belgium, Belgium, May 2014. ICST (Institute for Computer Sciences, Social-Informatics and Telecommunications Engineering) (2014)
6. Gargantini, A., Terzi, F., Zambelli, M., Bonfanti, S.: A low-cost virtual reality game for amblyopia rehabilitation. In: Proceedings of REHAB, the 3rd 2015 Workshop on ICTs for Improving Patients Rehabilitation Research Techniques (REHAB 2015), pp. 81–84, New York, NY, USA. ACM (2015)
7. Rastegarpour, A.: A computer-based anaglyphic system for the treatment of amblyopia. Clin Ophthalmol. **5**, 1319–1323 (2011). doi:10.2147/opth.s25074. epub 2011 sep 16 2011 (Auckland, N.Z.)
8. Statt, N.: Facebook has oculus, Google has cardboard (2015). http://www.cnet.com/news/facebook-has-oculus-google-has-cardboard/. Accessed 7 Oct 2015
9. Suttle, C.M.: Active treatments for amblyopia: a review of the methods and evidence base. Clin. Exp. Optometry **93**, 287–299 (2010)

10. To, L., Thompson, B., Blum, J.R., Maehara, G., Hess, R.F., Cooperstock, J.R.: A game platform for treatment of amblyopia. IEEE Trans. Neural Syst. Rehabil. Eng. **19**(3), 280–289 (2011)
11. Vitali, A., Facoetti, G., Gargantini, A.: An environment for contrast-based treatment of amblyopia using 3D technology. In: International Conference on Virtual Rehabilitation 2013, August 26–29, 2013 in Philadelphia, PA, USA (2013)
12. Waddingham, P.E., Cobb, S.V., Eastgate, R.M., Gregson, R.M.: Virtual reality for interactive binocular treatment of amblyopia. In: The Sixth International Conference on Disability, Virtual Reality and Associated Technologies (2006)
13. Webber, A.L., Wood, J.: Amblyopia: prevalence, natural history, functional effects and treatment. Clin. Exp. Optometry **88**(6), 365–375 (2005)
14. Wei, H., Zhao, Y., Dong, F., Saleh, G., Ye, X., Clapworthy, G.: A cross-platform approach to the treatment of ambylopia. In: 2013 IEEE 13th International Conference on Bioinformatics and Bioengineering (BIBE), pp. 1–4. IEEE (2013)

Interactive Kinect-Based Rehabilitation Framework for Assisting Children with Upper Limb Cerebral Palsy

Mohammad I. Daoud$^{(\boxtimes)}$, Rami Alazrai, Abdullah Alhusseini, Dima Shihan,
Ekhlass Alhwayan, Dhiah el Diehn I. Abou-Tair, and Talal Qadoummi

School of Electrical Engineering and Information Technology,
German Jordanian University, Amman 11180, Jordan
{mohammad.aldaoud,rami.azrai,a.alhusseini,d.alshihan,
e.alhwayan,dhiah.aboutair,t.qadoummi}@gju.edu.jo

Abstract. The use of computer games as adjunct to conventional cerebral palsy (CP) rehabilitation provides a promising approach to actively engage CP children in physical therapy exercises. This chapter provides a summary of previous studies that incorporated computer games for CP rehabilitation. Moreover, a comprehensive game-based rehabilitation framework is presented to enable CP children to actively participate in upper-limb physical exercises. The framework design is based on five features that aim to achieve enjoyable and effective game-based physical exercises for complementing conventional CP rehabilitation. A prototype implementation of the framework is developed, which includes three Kinect-based games that target upper-limb excesses. The prototype implementation was employed in the rehabilitation of three CP patients, and the preliminary results suggest the feasibility of the framework for complementary CP rehabilitation. The chapter also discusses some design challenges that are being tackled to continue the development of the comprehensive rehabilitation framework along with proposed solutions.

Keywords: Cerebral palsy · Serious games · Computer games for physical therapy · Physical rehabilitation · Microsoft Kinect motion sensor · Motion capture

1 Introduction

Cerebral palsy (CP) describes a set of motion disorders that are responsible for human physical disability, particularly in body movements and muscle coordination [24]. According to the Centers for Disease Control and Prevention [1], CP is the most common motor disorder of childhood. The study by Winter *et al.* [26] indicated that 500,000 infants are affected by CP in the United States. The prevalence rate of CP in Europe is 2.08 per 1000 live births [18]. In general, CP is caused by non-progressive brain disturbances or malformation that takes

© Springer International Publishing AG 2017
H.M. Fardoun et al. (Eds.): REHAB 2015, CCIS 665, pp. 126–140, 2017.
https://doi.org/10.1007/978-3-319-69694-2_12

place while the fetal or infant brain is under development. Therefore, the CP disorders are permanent and non-progressive.

Children with CP suffer from various motor disorders that cause problems in the control and range of body movements [23]. These limitations affect the capability of CP children to perform daily-life activities, such as object grasping and manipulation [22], posture [30], and gait [6]. Currently, there is no specific therapy for the insults in brain that cause CP motor disorders [23]. In fact, the management and treatment of children with CP is mainly focused on participating in rehabilitation schemes that aim to improve weak muscles, enhance mobility skills, encourage functional independence, and reduce the development of secondary problems such as muscles contractions and skeletal deformations [23]. One effective CP rehabilitation scheme is the active participation in repetitive physical exercises. However, limited percentage of individuals with motor disabilities participates regularly in the exercises as recommended [28]. The reduced patient's motivation is often cited as a barrier to carry out the physical exercises on regular basis [20]. Furthermore, the number of exercises carried out in a regular therapy session is lower than the recommended number of daily exercises [19]. Other factors might also contribute to the reduced physical activity of children with CP, such as the limited access to equipment and the low availability of exercise instructors [14]. Therefore, the physical activities performed by CP children at home in an exciting and enjoyable environment provide an important complementary to conventional rehabilitation programs.

One promising approach to actively engage CP children in physical therapy exercises in an exciting and enjoyable environment is to use computer games as a complementary rehabilitation technology. In this context, serious games, which are games designed with a primary focus other than entertainment, such as rehabilitation, can be employed to increase the motivation of CP children and promote their physical activity [7,16]. In addition, commercial computer games can also be adopted for CP rehabilitation [32]. In fact, the recent advances in computer games technology, including the use of low-cost high-performance motion sensors, has the potential to enable the development of improved and powerful game-based rehabilitation tools for CP children.

In this chapter, we provide a summary of previous studies that addressed the development and adoption of computer games for CP rehabilitation. Moreover, a comprehensive game-based rehabilitation framework is proposed to actively engage children with CP in upper-limb physical exercises. The design of the framework is based on five key features for achieving supplementary rehabilitation exercises that effectively complement conventional rehabilitation programs. These features are: personalized game-based exercises that match the needs and capabilities of the CP patient, meaningful play [9], challenge adaptation [9], accurate evaluation of the patient's ability to perform the exercise targeted by the game, and enabling the physical therapist to monitor the progress of the CP patient over time. The implementation of the framework has been achieved by employing a Microsoft Kinect motion sensor to track the joints of the patient. The feasibility of the proposed framework has been demonstrated by developing a prototype implementation that incorporates three Kinect-based computer games for upper-limb CP physical exercises. The chapter also discusses some design challenges that are being tackled to continue the development of the comprehensive rehabilitation framework along with proposed solutions. These challenges include the human activity representation needed to automatically and accurately evaluate the patient's ability to perform the targeted game-based physical exercises, the capability of achieving group-based games to improve the social interaction of the CP patient, and the parallel computing resources needed to run the framework in real-time. A preliminary version of this work has appeared in [13], which included a limited review of the game-based rehabilitation of CP children and a brief description of the framework, without describing the framework design challenges and the proposed solutions. Moreover, the games described in the preliminary version were implemented using an older version of Microsoft Kinect.

The remainder of the chapter is organized as follows. Section 2 provides the literature review. Section 3 describes the five features of the framework and the proposed framework architecture. Furthermore, this section presents the prototype implementation of the framework along with preliminary testing and validation to evaluate its performance. The design challenges and the proposed solutions are described in Sect. 4. Finally, the conclusion and future directions as well as the acknowledgments are provided in Sect. 5.

2   Literature Review

Previous studies have suggested the use of computer games to actively engage CP children in the planned physical exercises and improve their motivation [7, 16]. In general, there are two approaches to integrate computer games in CP rehabilitation. In the first approach, commercial computer games are used as supplementary treatment for CP children. The second approach is to employ customized games that are specifically designed for CP rehabilitation.

The majority of the studies that involved commercial off-the-shelf games are focused on the use of the Nintendo Wii^{TM} technology (Nintendo Co. Ltd., Kyoto, Japan). For example, Winkels *et al.* [32] studied the effect of training CP children using commercial Nintendo Wii^{TM} sport games. The study concluded that the performance of daily life activities for CP children was improved after the training. Another instance of this approach is the pilot-study that was conducted by Gordon *et al.* [15] to investigate the visibility of using the Nintendo Wii^{TM} as a rehabilitation tool for children with CP. The interventions included a group of CP children who were trained using Wii Sports Boxing, Baseball, and Tennis games. The study indicated that the Nintendo Wii might provide a viable rehabilitation tool for children with CP, but clinical trials are needed to assess the effectiveness of this technology for improving the gross motor function. Jelsma *et al.* [17] used the Nintendo Wii Fit^{TM} for training children with spastic hemiplegic CP. The results indicated improvements in the patients' motivation and balance. Some researchers have also investigated the use of other commercial computer game technologies. For instance, Sandlund *et al.* [27] conducted a study in which children with CP were asked to practice with a Sony PlayStation2 (Sony, Tokyo, Japan) equipped with the EyeToy: Play 3 game set. This set includes 20 motion interactive games that are mainly focused on upper-extremity movements. The study suggested that training children with CP using motion interactive games has the potential to enhance arm motor control. Generally, the use of the off-the-shelf computer games for CP rehabilitation has the advantage of achieving high-quality game-playing experience using reduced costs. However, most commercial computer games are designed and developed for entertaining and promoting the physical activity of normal persons from the public. Therefore, the application of many commercial computer games for rehabilitation might be limited due to several factors, including the high-level of complexity and difficulty of the game, the limited game accessibility options that prevent the patient from playing the game, and the inability of assisting the progress of the patient based on the statistics provided by the game [5].

Many systems that include specifically-designed games and programs for CP rehabilitation employ virtual reality and motion tracking systems. For instance, in the study by Bryanton *et al.* [8], the effectiveness of virtual reality exercises for children with CP was compared with conventional exercises. The virtual reality exercises were carried out using the Interactive Rehabilitation and Exercise System (GestureTek, Ottawa, Ontario, Canada). In this system, the picture of the participant was recorded and integrated within a virtual environment that includes virtual objects displayed on a monitor. The participant performed the exercises by interacting with the virtual objects. The results suggested that virtual reality can enhance the effectiveness and excitement of physical exercises for children with CP. Chen *et al.* [11] developed a home-based virtual cycling training program to support lower-limb muscle strengthening in children with CP. In this program, the cycling exercises were performed using the Eloton Sim-Cycle Virtual Cycling System (Eloton, Inc., NV, USA) that incorporates an adaptive stationary cycling machine and a virtual reality environment for guiding the participants through virtual exercises. The study demonstrated that the virtual cycling training program can improve knee muscle strength in children with CP. It is worth noting that the systems that employ virtual reality usually involve high costs and require specialized equipment, which might limit their wide application for CP rehabilitation.

One attractive approach to build interactive, customized, game-based exercises for CP rehabilitation is to employ the Microsoft Kinect motion tracking sensor (Microsoft Corporation, Redmond, Washington, USA). The Kinect tracking sensor employs infrared depth sensing technology and an RGB camera along with sophisticated computational algorithms to construct a 3D map of the anatomical body landmarks, including body joints, at rates close to real-time [29]. Chang *et al.* [10] employed the Microsoft Xbox 360 Kinect^{TM} tracking sensor to develop a CP rehabilitation system that supports three degrees of freedom in upper-limb exercises. The system enabled the physical therapists to define a limited set of basic rehabilitation movements based on the motor impairment level of the patient.

The Kinect sensor was employed to track the body joints and calculate the accuracy of performing the rehabilitation movements. In another study by Roy *et al.* [25], a Kinect sensor was integrated with computer games to enable people with motor disabilities, including CP, to perform rehabilitation exercises in an exciting environment. In this system, a set of rehabilitation exercises were implemented in the form of Kinect-based mini-games that target specific limb motion problems. The patient interacted with the games through the Kinect sensor, which tracked the 3D motion of body joints. The score of the patient in each game was recorded and communicated to the doctor via a cloud-based logging system. Luna-Oliva *et al.* [21] conducted an interesting preliminary study to evaluate the possibility of using computer game exercises developed based on the Microsoft Xbox 360 Kinect^{TM} sensor to support conventional rehabilitation for children with CP. The results of this study suggested that the game-based treatment protocol, as adjunct to the conventional CP rehabilitation, has the potential to improve the patient's balance and quality of activities of daily living (ADL). The study also indicated that further investigations are required to evaluate the potential benefits of using Kinect-based computer games as complementary for conventional CP rehabilitation. The three studies described above demonstrate the feasibility of using Kinect-based computer games to enable low-cost, enjoyable motor rehabilitation systems that complement conventional physical rehabilitation exercises.

The previous studies that employed the Microsoft Kinect sensor for CP rehabilitation were mainly focused on the design and development of computer games that target specific body parts and evaluate their rehabilitation capabilities. In fact, there is a need to develop a comprehensive game-based rehabilitation framework that enables the physical therapist to coordinate, monitor, and supervise the CP rehabilitation process achieved using the Kinect-based game exercises and customize the games based on the capabilities and performance of the patient.

3   The Comprehensive Game-Based Rehabilitation Framework

In this section, we present a comprehensive game-based rehabilitation framework to supplement conventional upper-limb CP rehabilitation programs. The framework is based on five key features that aim to improve the effectiveness of game-based CP rehabilitation, motivate the patient to participate actively in the game-based physical exercises, enable the physical therapist to coordinate and monitor the rehabilitation process, and achieve effective monitoring of the performance of the CP patient. This section presents the five features and the architecture of the proposed CP rehabilitation framework. Then, a prototype implementation of the framework is introduced, which incorporates three Kinect-based games for upper-limb CP rehabilitation. Finally, preliminary testing and validation of the proposed framework are provided.

3.1   Features of the Proposed Rehabilitation Framework

Five features are identified to improve the effectiveness of the proposed rehabilitation framework and to enhance the patient's motivation to participate regularly in the game-based physical exercises. These features are described below:

1. **Personalized rehabilitation exercises:** The framework will incorporate a large set of computer games, such that each game targets a specific upper-limb exercise. This diverse set of games, which will be designed under the supervision of experienced physical therapists, will cover a wide spectrum of physical exercises. For each CP case, the physical therapist can prescribe a group of games that meets the requirements and capabilities of the patient.

2. **Meaningful play:** Burke *et al.* [9] reported a game design principle, called meaningful play, for achieving effective game-based stroke rehabilitation. Meaningful play implies that the feedback of the player's actions during the gameplay should be conveyed to the player in a clear, meaningful, and consistent manner. The concept of meaningful play will be employed in the proposed CP rehabilitation framework to enable the patient to understand the objectives of the game and measure his progress in accomplishing these objectives over time. The feedback can be delivered to the patient in several formats, such as aural and visual formats. Moreover, progress bars and game scores can be employed to deliver the feedback.

3. **Challenge adaptation:** Another design principle that have been reported by Burke *et al.* [9] for game-based stroke rehabilitation is challenge. This principle can also be applied for CP rehabilitation. The challenge principle refers to the adaptation of the difficulty level of the game based on the needs of the patient. Such an adaptation of the game difficulty is crucial since CP patients vary in their motor capabilities and game playing skills. Moreover, at the beginning of playing a game, the player requires low difficulty level due to his limited familiarity with the game. At a later stage, the player becomes familiar with the game, and hence a higher difficulty level is needed to keep the game challenging and interesting for the player. The physical therapist, who can evaluate the physical and cognitive abilities of the patient, will be involved in the configuration and modification of the game difficulty level to meet the abilities of the patient.

4. **Accuracy of performing the game exercise:** As mentioned above, each game will be designed to target a specific upper-limb physical exercise. The accuracy of performing the exercise will be evaluated by comparing the body movements performed by the player with the corresponding correct movements of the exercise. The body movements during the exercise will be tracked using a motion tracking system.

5. **Monitoring patient's progress:** The proposed framework will maintain a record of the patient's performance over time. The recorded performance data will mainly include a log of the patient's accuracy of performing the game exercise. This record will be provided to the physical therapist via the cloud to enable him to track the progress of the patient.

3.2   The Proposed Framework Architecture

The proposed rehabilitation framework is comprised of two main components: the central system that runs on the cloud, denoted as the cloud, and the patient's local system. Figure 1 illustrates the components of the proposed framework. The cloud is responsible for storing the latest versions of all games. Moreover, for each game, the cloud stores the body movements recommended by the physical therapist to accurately perform the physical exercise targeted by the game. Each patient will have a personal account on the cloud. This account stores the personal information of the patient, the set of games prescribed to the patient by the physical therapist, the customized configurations of the prescribed games as set by the physical therapist, and a log of the patient's performance. Furthermore, the cloud provides a web-based interface that allows the physical therapist to prescribe and configure games to the patients and view their performance progress.

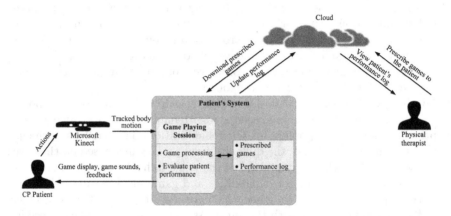

Fig. 1. The design of the proposed rehabilitation framework. The Microsoft Kinect is used to track the movements of the patient.

The patient's local system is composed of a personal computer connected to the cloud. The computer is connected to a motion tracking system for monitoring the 3D motion of the patient during the gameplay. The motion tracking system employed in this study is the Microsoft Kinect for Windows v2. The games prescribed by the physical therapist are downloaded from the cloud to the patient's local system. Each time the patient starts one of the prescribed games, all the processing of the game is performed by the local system. Moreover, the patient interacts with the game via the Kinect sensor. To evaluate the ability of the patient to perform the physical exercise targeted by the game, the movements of the patient's body joints during the gameplay are compared with the recommended body motions associated with the game. In addition, a log of patient's progress over time is stored in the patient's local system and uploaded to the cloud. During the gameplay, several performance feedback indicators, such as the game score and progress bars, are displayed on the screen. Moreover, at the end of the game, a report about the patient performance during the gameplay is displayed.

As the performance of the patient improves over time, the patient can send a request to upgrade the difficulty level of the game. This request is passed via the cloud to the physical therapist, who can approve or decline the patient's request. It is recommended that the physical therapist communicates directly with the patient before approving or declining his request.

3.3   Prototype Implementation of the Framework

During the development of the current version of the framework, we have worked with a specialized physical therapy center (Al Hussein Society Jordan Center for Training and Inclusion, Amman, Jordan[1]) to design and build three Kinect-based games that target upper-limb exercises. These games are brick breaker, tennis, and face parts that incorporate physical exercises for horizontal shoulder adduction/abduction, shoulder extension/flexion, and hand stability, respectively. Figure 2 shows sample images of the three games. The three targeted exercises along with the matching games are described as follows:

1. **Horizontal shoulder adduction and abduction:** This exercise is designed to enhance the degree of shoulder abduction and adduction of the patient. The patient in this exercise is asked to move his arm rightward and leftward while stretching the arm as far as possible. We implemented this exercise through the bric breaker game (see Fig. 2a). In this game, the player must break a wall of bricks through deflecting a bouncing ball with a paddle. The CP patient moves his arm horizontally (with some inclination at the shoulder) to control a paddle. The arm of the patient has to be stretched in a straight manner during the gameplay. The patient gains one point each time he hits a brick. The patient advances to a new level when all the bricks have been destroyed. The game ends when the patient fails to deflect the bouncing ball for three times. At the end of the game, the score of the patient is recorded and displayed on the screen. In addition, the deviation between the movements of the patient's arm and the recommended exercise arm movements throughout the gameplay is recorded.

2. **Shoulder extension and flexion:** This exercise is designed to enhance the degree of shoulder extension and flexion of the patient. The patient in this exercise is asked to move his arm upward and downward while stretching the arm as far as possible. This exercise has been implemented as a computer tennis game that simulates ground tennis (see Fig. 2b). The tennis game is designed to improve the state of the elbow and shoulder joints by engaging the patient in simple vertical motions of the arm. The patient in this game plays against a computer-controller opponent. Both the patient and the computer-controller player can move their paddles vertically to hit the ball back and forth. A player gains a point if the opponent player fails to return the ball.

---

[1] http://ahs.org.jo/.

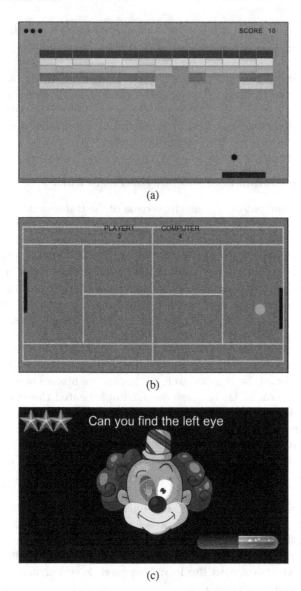

Fig. 2. Sample images of the (a) Brick breaker, (b) Tennis, and (c) Face parts games.

The player that reaches eleven points before the other wins the game. The ball speed is configured by the physical therapist based on the abilities of the patient.

3. **Hand stability:** This exercise is designed to enhance the patient's ability to stabilize his hands. The patient is asked to move his hand toward a specific object. Then, the patients will have to station his hand over that object for

a predetermined period of time. For the purpose of this exercise, we have implemented a game called face parts (see Fig. 2c). In this game, a clown face is displayed on the screen and the user is asked to find a specific part of the face (for example, find the left eye, right eye, etc.) within a specific time window. Then, the patient has to hold his hand over the face part for a given time period. The time period is initially set to three seconds and can be adjusted by the physical therapist. Each time the patient successfully finds a specific face part, a crowd cheer sound effect is played to encourage the patient and a star is displayed at the top left side of the screen to indicate gaining a point. The gameplay ends when the player fails to find the face part within the predefined time period for three times. At the end of the gameplay, the game score is displayed on the screen to indicate the number of face parts that have been correctly identified.

3.4 User Testing and Validation

In order to demonstrate the feasibility of the proposed framework to enable complementary CP rehabilitation, we have tested our framework with two sets of users:

1. **Healthy subjects:** Testing with healthy subjects enabled us to measure the performance of the framework, including the operation of the games, the ability to calculate the scores correctly, and the recording of the log file that stores user's performance, in a controlled environment. Figure 3 provides a sample image of a healthy subject during a gameplay of the face parts game.

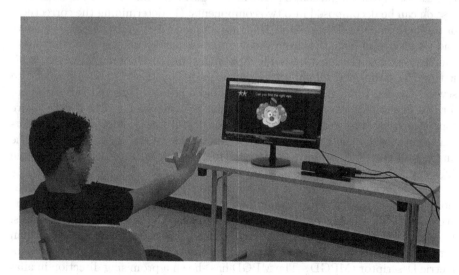

Fig. 3. Healthy subject playing the face parts game which realizes the hand stability exercise.

2. **CP patients:** In order to evaluate the performance of the proposed rehabilitation framework, we have stored the three games on the Microsoft Azure Cloud Service and made them available for three CP patients at the Al Hussein Society Jordan Center for Training and Inclusion. The three patients have downloaded the games on their local computer systems. In addition to the three games, we have built a feedback system to enable the physical therapist to track the progress of the CP patients. The feedback is communicated from the local computer of each patient to the smartphone of the physical therapist via the cloud. The three patients have participated in the three games several times. They have indicated that the three games enabled them to participate in physical therapy exercises in an exciting and enjoyable environment. Moreover, the physical therapist suggested that the proposed framework provides an effective supplementary system to complement conventional rehabilitation programs.

4   Design Challenges and Solutions

4.1   Human Activity Representation and Performance Evaluation

In general, CP rehabilitation exercises can be viewed as human activities that involve spatiotemporal movements of body-parts such as hands, arms, feet, legs, torso, and head. Human activities can be defined in terms of the pose and motion profiles of the body parts, the relative temporal ordering, and the interdependency of moving body-parts [4]. A CP rehabilitation system heavily relies on the representation of the human activity for evaluating the performed rehabilitation exercises and assessing the progress of the patient's treatment. In this context, the assessment of the patient's performance during a game-based rehabilitation session can be decomposed into two components: (1) determining the correctness of the performed exercises, and (2) identifying incorrect body-parts movements and the degree of deviation from the designated motions during a rehabilitation exercise session. Having that said, developing an automated system for evaluating the performed rehabilitation exercises is considered challenging due to several factors. First, moderate inter-personal and intra-personal variations are formed in the performed patient's activities. Second, human activities that are represented as a sequence of video images or depth images, such as the data format employed by the Kinect sensor, are high-dimensional data. Therefore, the analysis of this data requires a suitable spatiotemporal representation scheme that can reduce the dimensionality of the input domain.

This brings us to the point that the more relevant spatiotemporal information that is encapsulated in the human activity representation, the higher the accuracy in identifying incorrect activities during CP rehabilitation exercises. Recently, Alazrai *et al.* [2–4] have proposed an anatomical-plane-based human activity representation for analyzing human activities, called Motion-Pose Geometric Descriptor (MPGD). The MPGD has shown a promising direction in analyzing human activities that involve both one and two persons, such as human-human interactions [4], elderly fall detection [3], and elderly fall prediction [2].

Due to the improved capability of the MPGD to represent and analyze human activities, we are currently extending the current implementation of the framework to adopt the MPGD for representing the activities of the CP patients during upper-limb CP rehabilitation exercises. In particular, the MPGD utilizes the Microsoft Kinect sensor to capture the upper limb activities of the patient. Since the proposed framework is focused on upper-limb exercises, the MPGD is modified to acquire and analyze the 3D locations of the following sixteen skeletal joints: hip center, spine, shoulder center, head, left (L)/right (R) hand, L/R wrist, L/R elbow, L/R shoulder, and L/R hip. Based on these skeletal joint positions, the modified MPGD incorporates two profiles describing the motion and the pose of the upper-limb human body-parts.

The first profile is the motion profile. This profile describes the motion of different body-parts with respect to three anatomical imaginary planes, namely, Sagittal plane (**SP**), Coronal plane (**CP**), and Transverse plane (**TP**) [31]. Specifically, the intersection of the anatomical planes divides the 3D-space around a human shoulder into eight octants, which allows to determine the motion direction of each of the 3D skeletal-joint points by identifying the octant in which its displacement vector falls. Furthermore, dividing the anatomical-planes into a number of bins, allows to assign a semantic meaning to the observed motion, such as rightward and downward. The second profile is the pose profile. This profile captures different arm poses via utilizing a qualitative geometric pose features, namely, angle-based features. For example, the analysis of the right arm movements can be performed based on the angle-based features to calculate the angles between: (1) the line that extends from the right shoulder to the right elbow and the three anatomical planes, and (2) the line that extends from the right shoulder to the right elbow and the line that extends from the right elbow to the right wrist.

The capability of the MPGD to capture the semantic meaning of the performed patient's activities during the game-based exercises enables the construction of a classifier that can recognize the different sub-activities of the patient and identify both the correct and incorrect movements. For example, a classifier can be trained to identify the time intervals of the exercise during which the patient was not stretching out his arm to the required level, and reflect that on the game score and the log of the patient's progress records.

4.2   Improving Patient's Social Interaction

The irregular patient's participation in the physical exercises is considered a major challenge in CP rehabilitation. The main reason behind this problem is the reduced patient's motivation. One possible direction to improve the motivation of the patient to participate in the physical exercises is to create social relationships with other CP patients by participating in group games. Specifically, group games that support multiple players enable the patient to interact with other CP patients during the gameplay via the local network or the Internet. Such a capability will enhance the social interaction of the CP patients.

Currently, we are investigating the possibility of extending the proposed framework to include a set of group games that allow the CP patient to collaborate and compete with other CP patients. However, the application of this feature requires intensive research due to the variations in the physical and cognitive abilities of the CP patients.

4.3 Enabling Real-Time Execution of the Comprehensive Rehabilitation Framework

The substantial computational complexity that results due to the concurrent run of the Kinect-based games and the patient's performance evaluation using the MPGD method might lead to long execution times on serial computers. Such a limitation might prevent the real-time execution of the proposed framework. To overcome this challenge, our team is planning to employ parallel computing resources to run the comprehensive rehabilitation framework in real time. In particular, two low-cost parallel computing approaches will be investigated. The first approach is to implement the framework to run on a graphics processing unit (GPU) using the Compute Unified Device Architecture (CUDA) library (http://www.nvidia.com/object/cuda_home_new.html). Such an approach has been successfully used to run computationally-intensive applications in real time [12]. The second approach is to use the parallel computing resources offered by multi-core processers. This solution does not involve additional costs since most current processors support multi-core technology.

5 Conclusion and Future Work

A comprehensive framework is proposed to enable children with upper-limb CP to participate actively in physical rehabilitation exercises. The framework complements conventional rehabilitation programs by providing the patient with a set of customized Kinect-based games, such that each game targets a specific upper-limb physical exercise. These games are prescribed by the physical therapist based on the needs and abilities of the patient. The framework supports five features that insure the effectiveness of game-based rehabilitation, encourage the patient to actively participate in the games, and enables the physical therapist to monitor the progress of the patient. The future directions are focused on continuing the development of the framework to fully support the five features. In particular, an effective performance assessment model is being implemented based on the MPGD to allow accurate evaluation of the patient's performance progress. Moreover, the framework will be extended to support multiple players to improve the social interaction of the patients and will be implemented on a parallel computer platform to run in real time. The proposed framework will be made available to CP patients in different rehabilitation centers. Extended analysis will be carried out to evaluate the capability of the framework to complement conventional CP rehabilitation programs.

Acknowledgments. The authors acknowledge Al Hussein Society - Jordan Center for Training and Inclusion, Amman, Jordan for their support to design and develop the CP rehabilitation framework.

References

1. Centers for Disease Control and Prevention. http://www.cdc.gov/ncbddd/cp/index.html. Accessed 15 May 2016
2. Alazrai, R., Mowafi, Y., Hamad, E.: A fall prediction methodology for elderly based on a depth camera. In: 37th Annual International Conference of the IEEE Engineering in Medicine and Biology Society (EMBC), pp. 4990–4993, August 2015
3. Alazrai, R., Zmily, A., Mowafi, Y.: Fall detection for elderly using anatomical-plane-based representation. In: 36th Annual International Conference of the IEEE Engineering in Medicine and Biology Society (EMBC), pp. 5916–5919, August 2014
4. Alazrai, R., Mowafi, Y., Lee, C.G.: Anatomical-plane-based representation for human-human interactions analysis. Pattern Recognit. **48**(8), 2346–2363 (2015)
5. Annema, J.H., Verstraete, M., Abeele, V.V., Desmet, S., Geerts, D.: Videogames in therapy: a therapist's perspective. In: 3rd International Conference on Fun and Games, pp. 94–98, September 2010
6. Ballaz, L., Plamondon, S., Lemay, M.: Ankle range of motion is key to gait efficiency in adolescents with cerebral palsy. Clin. Biomech. **25**(9), 944–948 (2010)
7. Bonnechere, B., Jansen, B., Omelina, L., Da Silva, L., Mougeat, J., Heymans, V., Vandeuren, A., Rooze, M., Van Sint Jan, S.: Use of serious gaming to increase motivation of cerebral palsy children during rehabilitation. Eur. J. Paediatr. Neurol. **17**, S12 (2013)
8. Bryanton, C., Bosse, J., Brien, M., Mclean, J., McCormick, A., Sveistrup, H.: Feasibility, motivation, and selective motor control: virtual reality compared to conventional home exercise in children with cerebral palsy. Cyberpsychol. Behav. **9**, 123–128 (2006)
9. Burke, J.W., McNeill, M.D.J., Charles, D.K., Morrow, P.J., Crosbie, J.H., McDonough, S.M.: Optimising engagement for stroke rehabilitation using serious games. Vis. Comput. **25**, 1085–1099 (2009)
10. Chang, Y.J., Han, W.Y., Tsai, Y.C.: A kinect-based upper limb rehabilitation system to assist people with cerebral palsy. Res. Dev. Disabil. **34**, 3654–3659 (2013)
11. Chen, C., Hong, W., Cheng, H., Liaw, M., Chung, C., Chen, C.: Muscle strength enhancement following home-based virtual cycling training in ambulatory children with cerebral palsy. Res. Dev. Disabil. **33**, 1087–1094 (2012)
12. Chung, J., Daoud, M.I., Imani, F., Mousavi, P., Abolmaesumi, P.: GPU accelerated implementation of ultrasound radio-frequency time series analysis. In: Proceedings of SPIE, vol. 8320, pp. 83201I–83201I-7 (2012)
13. Daoud, M.I., Qadoummi, T., Abou-Tair, D.: An interactive rehabilitation framework for assisting people with cerebral palsy. In: Proceedings of the 3rd 2015 Workshop on ICTs for Improving Patients Rehabilitation Research Techniques, pp. 46–49 (2015)
14. Fowler, E.G., Kolobe, T.H., Damiano, D.L., et al.: Promotion of physical fitness and prevention of secondary conditions for children with cerebral palsy: section on pediatrics research summit proceedings. Phys. Therapy **87**, 1495–1510 (2007)
15. Gordon, C., Roopchand-Martin, S., Gregg, A.: Potential of the nintendo Wii™ as a rehabilitation tool for children with cerebral palsy in a developing country: a pilot study. Physiotherapy **98**, 238–242 (2012)

16. Howcroft, J., Klejman, S., Fehlings, D., Wright, V., Zabjek, K., Andrysek, J., Biddiss, E.: Active video game play in children with cerebral palsy: potential for physical activity promotion and rehabilitation therapies. Arch. Phys. Med. Rehabil. **93**(8), 1448–1456 (2012)

17. Jelsma, J., Pronk, M., Ferguson, G., Jelsma-Smit, D.: The effect of the nintendo Wii Fit on balance control and gross motor function of children with spastic hemiplegic cerebral palsy. Dev. Neurorehabil. **16**, 27–37 (2013)

18. Johnson, A.: Prevalence and characteristics of children with cerebral palsy in Europe. Dev. Med. Child Neurol. Null **44**, 633–640 (2002)

19. Kleim, J.A., Hogg, T.M., VandenBerg, P.M., Cooper, N.R., Bruneau, R., Remple, M.: Cortical synaptogenesis and motor map reorganization occur during late, but not early, phase of motor skill learning. J. Neurosci. **24**, 628–633 (2004)

20. Lloyd-Jones, D., Adams, R.J., et al.: Heart disease and stroke statistics-2010 update: a report from the american heart association. Circulation **121**, 46–215 (2010)

21. Luna-Oliva, L., Ortiz-Gutierrez, R.M., Cano-de la Cuerda, R., Piedrola, R.M., Alguacil-Diego, I.M., Sanchez-Camarero, C., Martinez Culebras Mdel, C., : Kinect Xbox 360 as a therapeutic modality for children with cerebral palsy in a school environment: a preliminary study. Neurorehabilitation **33**, 513–521 (2013)

22. McConnell, K., Johnston, L., Kerr, C.: Upper limb function and deformity in cerebral palsy: a review of classification systems. Dev. Med. Child Neurol. **53**(9), 799–805 (2011)

23. Papavasiliou, A.: Management of motor problems in cerebral palsy: a critical update for the clinician. Eur. J. Paediatr. Neurol. **13**(5), 387–396 (2009)

24. Rosenbaum, P., Paneth, N., Leviton, A., Goldstein, M., Bax, M., Damiano, D., Dan, B., Jacobsson, B.: A report: the definition and classification of cerebral palsy April 2006. Dev. Med. Child Neurol. **49**, 8–14 (2007)

25. Roy, A.K., Soni, Y., Dubey, S.: Enhancing effectiveness of motor rehabilitation using kinect motion sensing technology. In: Research in Developmental Disabilities, pp. 298–304 (2013)

26. Winter, S., Autry, A., Boyle, C., Yeargin-Allsopp, M.: Trends in the prevalence of cerebral palsy in a population-based study. Pediatrics **110**, 1220–1225 (2002)

27. Sandlund, M., Domellöfb, E., Gripa, H., Rönnqvistb, L., Hägera, C.K.: Training of goal directed arm movements with motion interactive video games in children with cerebral palsy - a kinematic evaluation. Dev. Neurorehabil. **17**, 318–326 (2014)

28. Shaughnessy, M., Resnick, B., Macko, R.: Testing a model of post-stroke exercise behavior. Rehabil. Nurs. **31**, 15–21 (2006)

29. Shotton, J., Fitzgibbon, A., Cook, M., et al.: Real-time human pose recognition in parts from single depth images. In: Proceedings of 2011 IEEE Conference on Computer Vision and Pattern Recognition, pp. 1297–1304 (2011)

30. Slaboda, J., Lauer, R., Keshner, E.: Postural responses of adults with cerebral palsy to combined base of support and visual field rotation. IEEE Trans. Neural Syst. Rehabil. Eng. **21**(2), 218–224 (2013)

31. Snell, R.S.: Clinical Anatomy by Regions, 9th edn. Lippincott Williams & Wilkins, Walters Kluwer, Philadelphia (2011)

32. Winkels, D.G.M., Kottink, A.I.R., Temmink, R.A.J., Nijlant, J.M.M., Buurke, J.H.: Wii^{TM}-habilitation of upper extremity function in children with cerebral palsy: an explorative study. Dev. Neurorehabil. **16**, 44–51 (2013)

Neuropsychological Predictors of Alcohol Abtinence Following a Detoxification Program

Bruno Bento[1,3(✉)], Jorge Oliveira[1,2], Fátima Gameiro[1,2], Rodrigo Brito[1,2], Pedro Gamito[1,2], Paulo Lopes[1,2], Diogo Morais[1,2], and Margarida Neto[3]

[1] EPCV/Lusophone University, Campo Grande, 376, Lisbon, Portugal
brunoricardobento@hotmail.com,
{jorge.oliveira,p2397,rodrigo.brito,pedro.gamito,p2209,
diogo.morais}@ulusofona.pt
[2] EPCV and COPELABS/Lusophone University, Campo Grande, 376, Lisbon, Portugal
[3] Casa de Saúde do Telhal, Mem-Martins, Portugal
margarida.neto@isjd.pt

Abstract. Alcohol dependence syndrome has been associated to disfunctions of the pre-frontal cortex, with a negative impact on several areas of cognitive functioning, such as attention, memory and learning, visual-spatial synthesis, executive functions, and psychomotor functions. These changes in turn contribute to the perpetuation of the addictive behavior. We report a study with 249 recovering alcoholics assessed with neuropsychological tests pre- and post-treatment at an alcoholism rehab clinic, with follow-up for abstinence 3 and 6 months after treatment. We found that 3-month abstinence was associated to speed of psychomotor processing, whereas 6-month abstinence was related with decision-making, (lack of) impulsivity, speed of psychomotor processing, and emotional adjustment.

Keywords: Alcoholism · Abstinence · Neuropsychological assessment · Predictors of abstinence

1   Introduction

Alcholic beverages have been produced and consumed for about 8000 years, but their consumption only became a public health problem from the industrial revolution onward, due to its mass sale [1]. Alcohol abuse is a progressive, chronic, and multifactor disease and public health issue. According to the World Health Organization (WHO) alcohol abuse is a lifestyle-related public health problem and alcohol is the most widely consumed drug in the World, being consumed by about two billion people [2]. In 2010, alcohol was responsible for 3.3% of deathers and 5.9% of working years lost; the European Union is the region of the world with highest per capita consumption (10.9 litres of alcohol per year) and worldwide, per capita consumption of over-15 year olds was 6.2 litres per year, or 13.5 grams per day; and males consume more than females [3].

© Springer International Publishing AG 2017
H.M. Fardoun et al. (Eds.): REHAB 2015, CCIS 665, pp. 141–149, 2017.
https://doi.org/10.1007/978-3-319-69694-2_13

1.1 Causes and Consequences of Alcoholism

Alcohol dependence syndrome (ADS) is a chronic multi-causal disease, including genetic, social, cultural, and psychological causes. At the genetic level, research has identified a mutant allele (ALDH2*2/*2) that functions as a buffer against the development of the symptoms of alcoholism by accelerating the metabolization of toxic acetic aldeid, an intermediary substance based on metabolization of ethyl alcohol by the organism that is responsible for the symptoms of acute alcoholic intoxication. Individuals with this allele are thus more disposed to drink alcohol in larger quantities and develop dependency [4]. Social and cultural causes of alcoholism refer to the availability of alcohol and with the cultural and social norms and attitudes towards alcohol, and psychological or personality factors may include low self-esteem, sensation-seeking, escape from pain, and unfavorable family relations [5].

Alcohol consumption enhances the neurotransmission of monoamines such as Dopamine (DA), norepinefrine (NE) e serotonine (5-HT) in synapses by blocking the uptake mechanism; the reinforcement effect of ethanol depends critically on DA, being implicated in the mesolimbic system [6]. Persistent stimulation of dopaminergic and serotinergic circuity, in particular in the aacumbens nucleus, has a motivational and emotional effect on alcohol addicts [7, 8]. Adaptative and enhanced activity of the 5-HT2 receptors under chronic presence of ethanol may contribute to alcohol abstinence syndrome when this is withdrawn [9].

1.2 Treatments for Alcoholism

Because ADS is a multifactorial disorder, its treatment should involve interventions at several levels: pharmacological, deep brain stimulation, or psychotherapeutic. Whatever the level of intervention, however, it will only be successful if alcoholics are in abstinence, which is the main goal of alcohol rehabilitation clinics.

Pharmacological intervention is mostly focused on alcohol abstinence syndrome (AAS), and uses medication such as dissulfiram that blocks the capacity to metabolize alcohol and produces nausea, naxeltrone that reduces pleasurable feelings produced by alcohol, and acamprosate that reduces alcohol craving, and more recently ondansetron and topiramato [10]. Research on the brain circuits that lead to alcoholism also opened up a path for Deep Brain Stimulation (DBS), use of this technique to treat alcoholism was hit upon by accident in 2007 as a by-product of a treatment for severe anxiety and depression, by stimulating the accumbens nucleus [11]. This technique has meanwhile been adopted for the treatment of several psychiatric disorders and addictions, including tobacco and alcohol [12–14]. Psychotherapy is also indispensable for alcoholics' ability to remain abstinent. Despite the fact that none of the many intervention methods has proven completely effective, they retain an important role in the psychological maturity and the social and family reinsertion of patients, through the establishment of strategies and essential goals for an effective treatment [15]. Finally, a variety of research has shown that cognitive stimulation is effective in the recovery of the cognitive abilities of alcoholics [16–24]. The strategy of cognitive stimulation is based on the repetition of tasks that aim to stimulate the plasticity that the brain has to adapt to demanding environmental circumstances [25].

1.3   Impact of Excessive Consumption of Alcohol at the Individual and Social Level

Excess consumption of alcohol can lead to alcohol use disorder (AUD), which is characterized in the DSM-V by: prioritization of drinking over other spheres of life; uncontrolled, excessive and recurrent drinking; increased tolerance to alcohol; symptoms of abstinence and relief of abstinence through further drinking; and by concurrent social and professional problems linked to alcohol abuse [26]. The negative effects of alcohol use on brain functions are evident from the literature; the most obvious effects are on the pre-frontal cortex. The chronic consumption of ethanol is associated to changes in memory and learning, in visual-spatial analysis and synthesis, in psychomotor speed, in executive functions, in decision-making, in impulsivity and psychomotor lentification and information processing, and in some can result in persistent pathologies of memory and in alcoholic dementia, such as the Wernike-Korsakov syndrome [17, 27, 28]. Alcoholism is also associated to impulsivity [29, 30]. Impulsive individuals have difficulty in postponing rewards or an immediate pleasure, and are unable to wait for and understand future behaviors [31]. Alcoholics tend to exhibit changes in their decision-making process and make choices that do not take into account their future consequences [28]. Faced with the dilemma of drinking or keeping abstinent, patients' choice of immediate pleasure and relief of symptoms is due to changes in the pre-frontal cortex that damage an efficient decision-making process; most addicts show reduced decision-making process, suggesting an insensibility to future consequences [32].

These deficits in ADS patients are positively correlated with consumption patterns (i.e. social drinkers vs. alcoholics) [33] and the consequences of ethanol consumption extend to the neurological dimension, in particular at the level of the pre-frontal cortex: functional and morphological changes have an effect on the reduction glucose and blood flow and in neuropsychological deficits in executive control, impulsivity and attention, which reveal themselves as a pathology of the frontal lobe and alcohol disorder [34]. In fact, over half of the patients in alcohol recovery programs show some level of deficits in abstract reasoning, executive functions, spatial abilities, learning, and memory [22].

Conversely, alcoholics with greater changes in frontal functions, namely in inhibitory control and working memory tasks, tend to have worse prognoses and a higher relapse frequency during recovery programs. This suggests that executive functions such as inhibitory control and working memory are essential to maintain a consistent abstinent behavior. Executive functions are also crucial to maintain and achieve life projects, follow conversations (socialize) and in general for a sustainable day-to-day functioning. Therefore, cognitive deficits in alcoholics are both cause and consequence of continuing dependency [17, 34]. Research also shows that frontal deficits in alcoholics have direct implications on the treatment itself, whether for the choice of strategy or for the prognose of patients [17, 27, 34, 35].

In previous studies [36] we have shown that cognitive training through serious games in recovering alcoholics can enhance the recovery of cognitive performance, namely mental flexibility. The current study is an extension of that work, in which we seek to identify neuropsychological variables that can predict abstinence in recovering alcoholics, refining the precision of prognoses for recovery with the use of neuropsychological assessment.

2   Method

2.1   Participants and Procedure

249 patients aged 27 to 73 (M^{age} = 48.63yrs, 80.3% male, with an average 11yrs of formal education) diagnosed with alcohol dependence syndrome and undergoing a detoxification program at a Portuguese private clinic were randomly recruited for this study. Most participants (97.1%) were Portuguese, slightly less than half (44.5%) were employed, and only a third (33.3%) were married. All patients followed a medication regime including Diazepam, Triapride, and vitamins, to minimize abstinence symptoms and a deregulation of complex B vitamins.

Post-treatment mortality from the study was 139 participants 3 months after the end of the treatment, but only 88 after 6 months. Telephone follow-up by the nursing team at the clinic explains this lower mortality after 6 months compared to 3 months.

Patients who agreed to participate and signed an informed consent form underwent a neuropsychological assessment during their first days of treatment, after being cleared of withdrawal symptoms by the local psychiatrist (last author). All the participants again underwent the neuropsychological treatment 4 weeks later at the end of their treatment. They were then invited to attend follow-up appointments with the neuropsychological team at the clinic 3 and 6 months after the end of the treatment. Participants who attended theses appointments underwent a number of tests – Iowa Gambling Test (IGT) for decision-making, the SCL-90-R for emotional adjustment and the UPPS+P impulsivity scale. Participants were asked about their possible consumption of alcohol after the end of their treatment and contacted by telephone by the nursing staff of the clinic. Data on abstinence were registered at 3 and 6 months and coded dichotomically (no relapse vs relapse) as well as in more detailed form (some relapse, lower or higher consumption compared to pre-treatment, etc.). About a third of the patients also underwent a cognitive stimulation program, but here we analyze the whole sample together.

2.2   Measures

Memory was assessed with the Wechsler Memory Scale (WMS) [37], which measures auditive learning memory, long-term retention, and working memory. In particular, working memory was assessed with the digit test (inverse order digit memory). *Mental flexibility* was assessed with the Wisconsin Card Sorting Test (WCST) [38], which is commonly used to assess executive functions, such as strategic planning, abstract thinking, and perseverant behaviors. *Decision-making* was assessed with the Iowa Gambling Task (IGT) [28], which is a measure commonly used in the framework of addictions to detect impulsive decision-making behaviors, as well as with the UPPS+P impulsivity measure [39, 40], which measures negative urgency, positive urgency, lack of premeditation, and lack of perseverance. *Emotional disadjustment* was measured with the SCL-90-R scale [41] que nos permitiu discriminar nove dimensões de desajustamento emocional: somatização, obsessões/compulsões, sensibilidade interpessoal, depressão ansiedade, hostilidade, ansiedade fóbica, ideação paranoide e o psicoticismo. *Depressive symptoms* were assessed with the Portuguese version Becks Depression Inventory II (BDI-II) [42, 43], which is a 21 multiple choice-item self-report scale.

3   Results

Simple correlation analyses indicate that regularity of consumption of alcohol is not very associated with cognitive performance, except for the Wechsler reverse numbers ($r = .17$) and the WCST number of conceptual answers measure ($r = .16$). However, we used a relatively conservative measure of alcohol consumption and this produced a ceiling effect, which may explain the low correlations.

Specific measures of all the neuropsychological tests (1st and 2nd assessments, i.e. pre and post-treatment) were entered as independent variables in a series of four multiple linear regression analyses (stepwise method) with both complete abstinence and frequency of consumption at two moments – treatment plus 3 months and treatment plus 6 months – as dependent variables.

Complete abstinence 3 months after treatment was predicted by the percentile of time spent on the Rey Complex Figure (RCF) copy, 2nd evaluation ($F(1, 45) = 5.89$; $p = .019$), explaining 9.6% of the variance. No other variable had an independent significant effect.

In contrast, three different independent variables predicted complete abstinence at 6 months, explaining 40.9% of total variance ($F(3,40) = 10,912$; $p < .001$). The first variable entered was percentile of time spent on the RCF copy, 1st evaluation, which alone explained 17.7% of the variance; the second was total score on the UPPS+P, 2nd evaluation, which explained an additional 11.9% of variance, and the third was the ICT Deck B Raw Score, 2nd evaluation, which predicted 11.3% of total variance (Table 1).

Table 1. Multiple linear regression between neuropsychological variables and complete abstinence after 6 months

Steps	Ivs	Total Adj R^2	B
1	RCF copy percentile time spent 1st evaluation	.177	−0,009
2	UPPS Total 2nd evaluation	.296	−0,009
3	IGT Deck B Raw Score 2nd evaluation	.409	−0,012

Frequency of consumption after 6 months was predicted by six independent variables, explaining 53.2% of the variance ($F(5, 35) = 10.095$; $p < .001$), which explained a total of 53.2% of the variance. The first variable entered was percentile of time spent on the copy of the Rey Complex Figure, which explained 13.6% of the variance, followed by total score on the UPPS+P, 2nd assessment, which explained 13.5% of the variance, the IGT Deck B raw score, 2nd assessment, explaining 13.6% of the variance, total score of the UPPS+P, which explained 15.4% of the variance, and general index of symptoms on the SCL-90, 2nd assessment, which explained 6.2% of the variance, and finally IGT net total raw score, 2nd assessment, which explained 4.5% of the variance (Table 2).

Table 2. Multiple linear regression between neuropsychological variables and frequency of consumption after 6 months

Steps	IVs	Total Adj R2	β
1	FCR copy percentile time spent 2nd evaluation	.135	.411
2	IGT Deck B Raw Score 2nd evaluation	.271	.978
3	UPPS Total 2nd evaluation	.425	.254
4	SCL-90 General symptoms index 2nd evaluation	.487	.331
5	IGT Net Total Raw Score 2nd evaluation	.532	.581

4 Discussion

In this chapter, we report a study in which we tested the relation between neuropsychological functions and abstinence after an alcohol rehabilitation treatment. As we expected, we found that regularity of consumption had an effect on most of the measures of neuropsychological functioning. We also found effects of cognitive performance on abstinence, indicating that cognitive functions are at the same time a consequence and a cause alcohol abuse.

As regards cognitive functions and abstinence, in general, we found strongest effects on abstinence and reduction of alcohol consumption at 6 months, and these were predicted most precisely by cognitive performance during the second assessment (post-detoxification treatment). Participants who remained abstinent after 6 months had shown better short-term memory, better indicators of mental flexibility, less complaints about sensorial interference and anxiety, and better scores on premeditation on the impulsivity scale. Post-treatment, predictors of relapse before 6 months were complaints over sensorial interference, phobic anxiety, depression, psychoticism, paranoid ideation, and symptoms of the emotional readjustment scale, greater positive urgency, lack of premeditation and lack of perseverance in the impulsivity scale, mental flexibility, and depressive symptoms.

Some of our results indicate that the speed of psychomotor systems and visual-constructive abilities is related to short-term abstinence (i.e. 3 months). Indeed, attention and speed problems can have negative impact on information learning during recovery, and thus negative consequences on the ability to choose abstinence. We also found that impulsivity control as measured by neuropsychological tests had an effect on abstinence.

What we have not analyzed in this chapter is the effect of cognitive stimulation on abstinence, even though a third of the sample underwent a cognitive stimulation rehab program. Cognitive stimulation has been found to be effective in recovering cognitive functions such as visual-constructive abilities, frontal functions, executive control, attention and mental flexibility, memory and learning, and psychomotor processing [16–24, 36]. These capabilities in turn have been related to the abstinence of alcoholic participants [17, 34, 36]. In the current sample we could not verify the direct effect of cognitive stimulation on post-treatment abstinence of participants. However, a cognitive stimulation strategy could contribute to indirectly to patients' abstinence [17, 27, 34, 35]. In future studies, the effects of cognitive stimulation on abstinence should be better clarified so as to develop a predictive model of the indirect action of stimulation, with the cognitive improvements that are produced by it, on abstinence.

Acknowledgments. The authors would like to thank Susana Carreiro for her contribution to the collection of the post-treatment sample.

References

1. Zampronio, A.: Prevenção ao uso de drogas. Uma Acção educativa. O caso de Jataizinnho – PR. Curitiba (2011)
2. Organização Mundial da Saúde: Neurociências: consumo e dependência de substâncias psicoativas - Resumo. OMS, Geneva (2004)
3. World Health Organization: Global Status report on alcohol and health (2014). http://www.who.int/substance_abuse/publications/global_alcohol_report/msb_gsr_2014_1.pdf?ua=1
4. Linneberg, A., Gonzalez-Quintela, A., Vidal, C., Jørgensen, T., Fenger, M., Hansen, T., Pedersen, O., Husemoen, L.: Genetic determinants of both ethanol and acetaldehyde metabolism influence alcohol hypersensitivity and drinking behaviour among Scandinavians. Clin. Exp. Allergy **40**(1), 123–130 (2010). doi:10.1111/j.1365-2222.2009.03398.x.v
5. Stuart, G.W., Laraia, M.T.: Enfermagem Psiquiátrica, 4th edn. Rio de Janeiro (2002)
6. Di Chiara, G.: The role of dopamine in drug abuse viewed from the perspective of its role in motivation. Drug Alcohol Depend. **38**, 95–137 (1995)
7. Di Chiara, G.: Alcohol and dopamine. Alcohol World Health Res. **21**, 108–113 (1997)
8. Stahl, S.: Mechanism of action of serotonin selective reuptake inhibitors. Serotonin receptors and pathways mediate therapeutic effects and side effects. J. Affect. Disord. **51**, 215–235 (1998). http://dx.doi.org/10.1016/S0165-0327(98)00221-3
9. Lovinger, D.: Alcohols and neurotransmitter gated ion channels: past, present and future. Naunyn-Schmiedeberg's Arch. Pharmacol. **356**(3), 267–282 (1997)
10. Andrade, A., Cruz, M.: Alcoolismo: recursos terapêuticos e agentes farmacológicos promissores. Jornal Brasileiro de Psiquiatria **54**(4), 270–276 (2005)
11. Kuhn, J., Lenartz, D., Huff, W., Lee, S., Koulousakis, A., Klosterkoetter, J., et al.: Remission of alcohol dependency following deep brain stimulation of the nucleus accumbens: valuable therapeutic implications? J. Neurol. Neurosurg. Psychiatry **78**(10), 1152–1153 (2007). doi:10.1136/jnnp.2006.113092
12. Christopher, P., Vassoler, F.: Deep brain stimulation for the treatment of addiction: basic and clinical studies and potential mechanisms of action. Psychopharmacology **229**(3), 487–491 (2013). doi:10.1007/s00213-013-3214-6
13. Kuhn, J., Grundler, T., Lenartz, D., Sturm, V., Klosterkotter, J., Huff, W.: Deep brain stimulation for psychiatric disorders. Deutsches Ärzteblatt International **107**(7), 105–113 (2010)
14. Sankar, T., Tierney, T., Hamani, C.: Novel applications of deep brain stimulation. Surg. Neurol. Int. **14**(3), s26–s33 (2012)
15. Heckmann, W., Silveira, C.: Dependência do álcool: aspectos clínicos e diagnósticos. In: Andrade, A., Anthony, J. (eds.) Álcool e suas conseqüências: uma abordagem multiconceitual, pp. 67–88. Editora Editora Manole Ltda, Brasil (2009)

16. Allen, D., Goldstein, G., Seaton, B.: Cognitive rehabilitaion of chronic alcohol abusers. Neuropsychol. Rev. **7**(1), 21–39 (1997)
17. Cunha, P., Novaes, M.: Avaliação neurocognitiva no abuso e dependência do álcool: implicações para o tratamento. Revista Brasileira de Psiquiatria **26**(1), 23–27 (2004)
18. Fals-Stewart, W., Lam, W.: Computer-assisted cognitive rehabilitation for the treatment of patients with substance use disorders: a randomized clinical trial. Exp. Clin. Psychopharmacol. **18**(1), 87–98 (2010). doi:10.1037/a0018058
19. Goldstein, G., Haas, G., Shemansky, J., Barnett, B., Salmon-Cox, S.: Rehabilitation during alcohol detoxication in comorbid neuropsychiatric patients. J. Rehabil. Res. Dev. **42**(2), 225–234 (2005)
20. Grohman, K., Fals-Stewart, W.: Computer-assisted cognitive rehabilitation with substance-abusing patients: effects on treatment response. J. Cogn. Rehabil. **21**(4), 10–17 (2003)
21. Gruber, S., Yurgelun-Todd, D.: Neuropsychological correlates of drug abuse. In: Kaufman, M. (ed.). Brain Imaging in Substance Abuse: Research, Clinical and Forensic Applications, Chap. 7, pp. 199–209. Humana Press, New Jersey (2001). doi:10.1007/978-1-59259-021-6_7
22. Oliveira, M., Laranjeira, R., Jaeger, A.: O estudo dos projectos cognitivos na dependência do álcool. Psicologia, Saúde e Doenças **3**(2), 205–2012 (2002)
23. Peterson, M., Patterson, B., Pillman, B., Battista, M.: Cognitive recovery following alcohol detoxification: a computerized remediation study. Neuropsychol. Rehabil. **12**(1), 63–74 (2002)
24. Yohman, T., Schaeffer, K., Parsons, O.: Cognitive training in alcoholic men. J. Consult. Clin. Psychol. **56**(1), 67–72 (1988)
25. Gamito, P., Oliveira, J., Lopes, P., Brito, R., Morais, D., Silva, D., Silva, A., Rebelo, S., Bastos, M., Deus, A.: Executive functioning in alcoholics following an mHealth cognitive stimulation program: randomized controlled trial. J. Med. Internet Res. **16**(4), e102 (2014). doi:10.2196/jmir.2923
26. American Psychiatric Association: Diagnostic and Statistical Manual of Mental Disorders, 5th edn. American Psychiatric Publishing, Arlington (2013)
27. Moselhy, H., Georgiou, G., Kahn, A.: Frontal lobe changes in alcoholism: a review of the literature. Alcohol Alcohol. **36**(5), 357–368 (2001). http://dx.doi.org/10.1093/alcalc/36.5.357
28. Bechara, A., Damásio, A.R., Damásio, H., Anderson, S.W.: Insensitivity to future consequences following damage to human prefrontal cortex. Cognition **50**(1–3), 7–15 (1994)
29. Dalley, J., Everitt, B., Robbins, T.: Impulsivity, compulsivity, and top-down cognitive control. Neuron Rev. **69**, 680–694 (2011)
30. Sun, H., Cocker, P., Zeeb, F., Winstanley, C.: Chronic atomoxetine treatment during adolescence decreases impulsive choice, but not impulsive action, in adult rats and alters markers of synaptic plasticity in the orbitofrontal cortex. Psychopharmacology **219**, 285–301 (2012)
31. Fisher, C., Fontes, M.: A impulsividade e o processo de tomada de decisão. Clínica Plenamente. Acedido a 17 de Maio de 2016 (2006). http://www.plenamente.com.br/artigo/181/-impulsividade-processo-tomada-decisaoclaudia-petlik.php#.Utw3FRCp1di
32. Bechara, A.: Decision making, impulse control and loss of willpower to resist drugs: a neurocognitive perspective. Nat. Neurosci. Neurobiol. Addict. **8**(11), 1458–1463 (2005)
33. Parsons, O.A.: Neurocognitive deficits in alcoholics and social drinkers: a continuum? Alcohol. Clin. Exp. Res. **22**(4), 954–961 (1998)
34. Blume, A., Marlatt, G., Schmaling, K.: Memory, executive cognitive function, and readiness to change drinking behavior. Addict. Behav. **30**(2), 301 (2005)

35. Rigoni, M., Oliveira, M., Susin, N., Sayago, C., Feldens, A.: Prontidão para mudança e alterações das funções cognitivas em alcoolistas. Psicologia em estudo **14**(4), 739–747 (2005). http://dx.doi.org/10.1590/S1413-73722009000400014

36. Oliveira, J., Bento, B., Gamito, P., Lopes, P., Brito, R., Morais, D., Gameiro, F.: Cognitive stimulation of alcoholics through VR-based Instrumental Activities of Daily Living. ACM Digital Library, pp. 14–17 (2015). doi:10.1145/2838944.2838948

37. Wechsler, D.: Wechsler Memory Scale - Third edition manual. Psychological Corporation, San Antonio (1987)

38. Heaton, R.K., Chelune, G.J., Talley, J.L., Kay, G.G., Curtiss, G.: Wisconsin card sorting test (WCST) — manual revised and expanded. Psychological Assessment Resources, Odessa (1993)

39. Whiteside, S.P., Lynam, D.R.: The five factor model and impulsivity: Using a structural model of personality to understand impulsivity. Personality Individ. Differ. **30**, 669–689 (2001)

40. Lopes, P., Oliveira, J., Brito, R., Gamito, P., Rosa, P., Trigo, H.: UPPS-P, versão portuguesa. Universidade Lusófona de Humanidades e Tecnologias, Lisboa (2013)

41. Derogatis, L.R., Savitz, K.L.: The SCL-90-R and the Brief Symptom Inventory (BSI) in Primary Care. In: Maruish, M.E. (ed.) Handbook of Psychological Assessment in Primary Care Settings, vol. 236, pp. 297–334. Lawrence Erlbaum Associates, Mahwah (2000)

42. Beck, A., Steer, R., Brown, G.: Manual for the Beck Depression Inventory II. Psychological Corporation, San Antonio (1996)

43. Martins, A., Coelho, R., Ramos, E., Barros, H.: Administração do BDI-II a adolescentes portugueses: resultados preliminares. Rev. Port. Psicossomática **2**(1), 123–132 (2000)

Virtual Rehabilitation on the Web: Analyzing and Improving Interaction in Postures Design

Félix Albertos-Marco[1]([✉]), José Antonio Fernández Valls[2], Víctor M.R. Penichet[1], María Dolores Lozano[1], and José A. Gallud[1]

[1] Computer Systems Department, University of Castilla-La Mancha, Albacete, Spain
{felix.albertos,victor.penichet,maria.lozano,
jose.gallud}@uclm.es
[2] Computer Science Research Institute (I3A), University of Castilla-La Mancha,
Albacete, Spain
josea.fernandez@uclm.es

Abstract. When interacting with interactive systems, users provide an input to the system and receive the corresponding output. On this cycle, there are translations between the components of the interactive process. But when using Web applications, translations can be affected due to the unique characteristics of the Web. Nowadays, and with the emergence of new interaction devices such as Microsoft Kinect which allows user movement to be captured, new approaches have appeared which facilitate the rehabilitation process. Web applications could be used on this process, for example, for designing postures or exercises. The creation of the postures may be complicated, involving a wide number of actions. If the physiotherapist does not feel comfortable using the rehabilitation system, it becomes cumbersome and hard to use. In this work we analyze how the interaction process of editing exercises in a virtual rehabilitation environment is affected when using Web applications. We propose the use local storage in a virtual rehabilitation environment based on the web to measure how it improves the interaction cycle and ultimately user usability and satisfaction.

Keywords: Rehabilitation · Exercise design · Virtual environment · Web applications · Local storage

1 Introduction

Interactive systems provide responses (outputs) according to the actions (inputs) provided by users. The use of the Internet has shifted not only the understanding on how software applications are deployed and used, but also how the interaction process is supported. It changed almost every area where software applications can be used. The advances in the standards of the web meant a revolution in the way of how Web applications are created and used.

In health-care contexts this movement helps democratizing health data management and widening its availability, having the potential to revolutionize telemedicine [5].

In rehabilitation process, patients need to be closely monitored by physiotherapists, who have to check that each exercise is performed correctly. Each individual patient

© Springer International Publishing AG 2017
H.M. Fardoun et al. (Eds.): REHAB 2015, CCIS 665, pp. 150–161, 2017.
https://doi.org/10.1007/978-3-319-69694-2_14

requires personalized attention. One goal in virtual rehabilitation environments is that patients are continuously monitored and guided in case they make mistakes. But from the point of view of the physiotherapists, one of the main goals is to customize the rehabilitation process to each patient. Therefore, the software has to allow them to create personalized exercises and control the correct perform of the therapy.

But when introducing Web applications in virtual rehabilitation environments new factors have to be taken into account. Due to the unique characteristics of Web applications, the creation of exercises in virtual environments may have some problems. As a result, usability may be affected. That is because one factor that has been previously neglected: Web applications are located remotely in Web servers. Therefore, there could be some delays when using them affecting the creation of postures.

To tackle with the drawbacks of using Web applications can be used several approaches. Nowadays, technologies allow the use of temporary storage in both the server and client side. But the last improvements on the Web allow managing local information in the browser. Moreover, these improvements allow the use offline Web applications. These approaches allow the improvement of user interaction.

In our work, which is an extended version of [3], we have found the main usability problems related with using Web applications in the design of postures in virtual rehabilitation environments. Then, we have proposed a solution for mitigating these problems.

This paper is structured as follow: Sect. 2 outlines related work; in Sect. 3 our system is described; Sect. 4 presents the evaluation; Sect. 5 contains a discussion; and finally Sect. 6 presents the conclusions and future work.

2   Related Work

In this section are presented rehabilitations applications related with our proposal as well as a previous approach of transforming an existent system to the Web. Finally, are outlined available techniques to manage local storage and offline interaction on Web applications.

2.1   Rehabilitation Applications

Due to the emergence of new interaction devices such as Microsoft Kinect which allows user movement to be captured, systems have appeared which facilitate the rehabilitation process. In this research field a series of virtual games has arisen: the so-called serious games, which attempt to motivate patients to carry out the rehabilitation process in a more effective, comfortable and friendly way [9, 10]. These systems allow the physiotherapist to choose the games their patients have to use. However, in the case of a patient needing a customized exercise, the specialist will not be able to design a new game because these systems are not developed for that purpose.

Rehabilitation software offers different games in which we can find specific exercises for a specific illness [7, 8]. Therefore, patients with other profiles cannot use these games.

Games, and the exercises in such games, are not fully adaptable to the different needs of every patient.

As a result, there are some systems which involve specialists in the development process of rehabilitation exercises [13]. If they need a specific exercise they are not able to design it by themselves. Therefore, they are forced to request developers to create a new application or to adapt an existent one, which could be slightly different.

But that is not the only issue when development applications for rehabilitation processes. The advance in Web technologies allows access to developed applications from mobile phones, computers or almost any device through the Internet, regardless of their physical location. In this way, there are some Web systems [12, 22] that aim to solve the problem of design rehabilitation exercises. However, these systems do not monitor or guide the user dynamically.

It is worthy to analyse another approach within the application of rehabilitation techniques. It consists in moving existent rehabilitation systems from desktop native applications to Web Environments. This approach was used by Ferriol with an existent system called play for Health (P4H) [14]. The incorporation of HTML5 [17] and Java-Script to P4H supposed a new client-side application that takes advantage of HTML5 features to overcome the limitations and functionalities that P4H had at that moment. As a result of Ferriol's work, the new version of P4H, Play for Health 2.0: Evolving P4H to a Web Environment Using HTML5 and JavaScript [5] was released.

Finally, there have been other approaches for improving user interaction with Web application in health-care environments. For example, McAllister [11] proposed an offline Web application using offline Web technologies to allow patients to save their readings offline without the need for network connection. This approach could be used in order to improve rehabilitation techniques using the Web.

2.2 Local Cache on Web Applications

Most of the approaches for cache management rely on server-side technologies such as proxy and server-side templates. However, technologies such as HTML5 and Web storage [19] make it possible to envisage new strategies for storing information from Web applications locally.

As stated above, storing information locally can be achieved using web storage. It introduces two mechanisms similar to HTTP session cookies for storing name-value pairs on the client side. The first is designed for scenarios where the user is carrying out a single transaction, but could carry out multiple transactions in different windows at the same time. The second storage mechanism is designed for storage that spans multiple windows. Despite the fact that Web storage is useful for storing pairs of keys and values, it does not provide in-order retrieval of keys, nor efficient searching over values or storage of duplicate values for a key. This technology could be used to store anything from user preferences or shopping cart information up to complex data structures. But there are ways to store and retrieve complex information structures locally. Web SQL Database [16] and Indexed Database API [18] allow the design of data schemas that are far more complex than simply using web storage. But Web SQL is no longer in active maintenance. Indexed Database provides a concrete API to perform advanced key-value data management that is at the heart of most sophisticated query processors. Furthermore, files can be also saved locally. The File API [20] allows the management of directories and files as in the operating system.

The World Wide Web Consortium (W3C) has recently proposed to integrate local storage management into their recommendations [17]. Indeed, the candidate recommendation of HTML5 fully integrates functions for local cache management and offline work using the Offline Web Applications technology [15], which was completely neglected in previous versions. Using HTML5's application Cache technology allows us to address the requirement of being always connected to use the web. However, one of the main issues with the Application Cache proposed in HTML5 is that there is no underlying model.

But the W3C is still developing specifications for dealing with the problems related to managing local information. One of the last and more promising efforts is the definition of the Service Workers [21]. This specification describes a method that could be used to manage Web applications in conjunction with the specifications presented above.

3   System Description

This section presents a brief description of the system with features and functions which are provided to physiotherapists to design the exercises in a personalized way. Lastly, the complete process to create an exercise is explained.

3.1   Brief Description of Our System

With the purpose of provide a system which allows therapists to design rehabilitation exercises to their patients, a Web-based system for designing and editing specific rehabilitation exercises has been developed. Three main features have to be taking into account when developing the system:

- Customization is an important feature of the system as it allows the therapist to adapt the exercises to the characteristics of each of their patients, in other words it offers not only customization, but personalization.
- Generated exercises could be monitored and guided by means of the Microsoft Kinect device.
- Provide access wherever the physiotherapist is located. In this way, access is possible from mobile phones, computers or any device through the Internet, regardless of physical location.

Using a 3D environment (Fig. 1), this system provides physiotherapists with a set of tools which allows them to design rehabilitation exercises and adapt them to the needs of the patient.

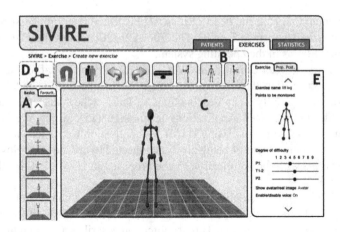

Fig. 1. Virtual Editor

The virtual environment (Fig. 1-C) shows a virtual space simulating a room whose proportions are the same according to the field of vision of Microsoft Kinect v2. It shows a skeleton comprising all the joints. The joints are basically the same joints used by Kinect v2. Matching these two models is natural, so the system can capture a Kinect posture as well as monitor in real time whether a patient's postures match the defined postures or not.

The x, y and z axes (Fig. 1-D) are very useful to move all the skeleton's joints together. If the control of one of the axes is moved, it is possible to see how the skeleton moves along this axis.

3.2 Rehabilitation Exercises

A rehabilitation exercise consists in adopting one specific posture without worrying about how this posture is achieved. Nevertheless, on many occasions the movement to reach one posture has its importance. Moreover, it is common to do complex rehabilitation exercises which are defined as a combination of postures and transitions between them. Furthermore, the system provides a set of customizable parameters (Fig. 1-E) such as joints to take into account, help text, difficulty level and voice activation.

In this environment designing postures is possible in two different ways:

- Manual interaction: specialist achieves the desired postures by interacting directly with the virtual environment;
- Motion-based interaction: using Microsoft Kinect the system captures the body posture of the specialist.

In the manual interaction, the therapist uses the virtual environment and interacts with a 3D skeleton. Therapists can create and design the desired postures. In order to design a posture, the physiotherapist has to drag and drop all the skeleton joints required to achieve the desired posture. Besides, he can use the different tool bars which are provided to complete the virtual space and to help the physiotherapist in the design process. These bars (Fig. 1-B) offer different tools such as redoing and undoing movements, choosing a specific perspective or designing the posture in a specific angle. With regard to making the design of postures process faster, a group of these are offered to the physiotherapist: basic and favourite postures (Fig. 1-A).

Additionally, the system offers the possibility of using Kinect for posture design. Kinect, with its motion-based interaction, enables the specialist to detect a user's joints and know their position. The location of each joint will be shown in the virtual environment so the physiotherapist can see the patient's movements in real time. Furthermore, the multiple voice commands can be used to operate the tools provided by the editor. It allows physiotherapists to conduct the process themselves. In first place, although they have activated the design tool with Kinect, not until the system recognizes the activate command for voice detection will the rest of the commands be available.

3.3 Detected Weaknesses

When using the manual interaction, we have detected some problems. Users do not feel really comfortable when using the system. They make mistakes because the system takes too much time to reflect the changes over the virtual editor. The delays in the interaction produced when designing postures make the system slow and users complain about this fact.

To illustrate how the interaction with the system is affected, the Fig. 2 presents the interaction model proposed by Abowd [1] and the translations between components: articulation, performance, presentation and observation. There, it is represented the interaction process between users and computers through their corresponding input and output channels. Each arc corresponds to a translation from one component to another.

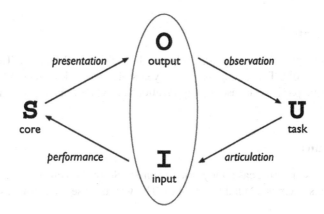

Fig. 2. Translations between components in the Interaction Model

When users are designing postures using the virtual editor they provide the input to the system (articulation). This input consists on the position of the joins that characterize the skeleton for each posture within the exercise. This input is translated (performance) to the language the system uses. Then, the system presents the updated posture translated (presentation) as the output of the system. Finally, the user shows the output (observation) provided by the system. The problem within the interactive system arises in the performance and the presentation translations. On these stages of the interaction cycle, the delays produced by the Web application makes the interaction cumbersome.

In order to assess this problematic and to solve it we perform an evaluation in two scenarios:

- Without using local storage. The system is used without any improvement.
- Using local storage. The system introduces an improvement consisting on using local storage to manage design posture creation. The communication with the remote server is performed in background without affecting the design process.

The use of local storage prevents the interaction delays in the performance and presentation translation presented in the Fig. 2. Other approaches could be considered, such as the use of model-based approaches for supporting offline interaction with Web applications [2]. But due to the characteristics of the virtual editor, these approaches are not feasible. They only support offline navigation, but not the interactive process of editing exercises in the presented editor.

In the next section is presented the evaluation addressing this problem in the described scenario.

4   Evaluation

To measure usability and user satisfaction in the developed system we have performed an evaluation. We expected quantitative and qualitative results to prove the feasibility of our approach.

4.1 Participants

The numbers of participants are 20. There are 12 males and 8 females. The youngest one has 21 years old. The average age is 23 years old. The oldest student has 37 years old. 100% of the participants use web applications daily. Participants were not paid for this activity.

4.2 Apparatus

The hardware used for the case study consists on an "Sony Vaio Pro 13" (2014 model)". The operating system is a Windows 8.1 Pro. The web browser is Chrome, version 43.

4.3 Design

The experiment follows a between-group design. 10 participants used the application without the improvement. The other 10 participants used the application with the improvement. In the evaluation we measure quantitative as well as qualitative indicators.

For quantitative indicator we use time meanwhile for qualitative indicator we use usability.

To carry out the experiment, users have to design a rehabilitation exercise. It is composed of four different postures which were shown on a paper. They had to use virtual environment and tools provided to perform the same postures and complete the exercise.

To measure quantitatively, we calculate two different aspects: the time to create a posture and the time to update it. First, each time user adds a posture, we register the time the system takes to create a posture, update the skeleton and add it to the postures list. Second, when user moves one of the skeleton's joints we register the time it takes for update the skeleton inside the virtual editor and updates the posture's image in the postures timeline.

4.4 Procedure

Each user is introduced to the system with a brief explanation on how it works explaining the different functions and tools. Then, the user starts to interact with the virtual editor without any additional information until he finishes the design of the exercise.

4.5 Results

Through the evaluation we get two metrics to analyse the improvement of our system: time and usability.

Regarding time, first we measure the time to create a posture. The Fig. 3 shows the time the system takes to create the postures without using local storage. The average time is 1398 ms.

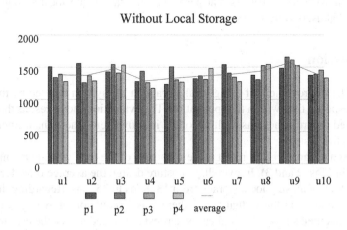

Fig. 3. Posture design: time without using local storage

In the other hand, the Fig. 4 shows the time the system takes to create the postures using local storage. In this case, the average time is 252 ms.

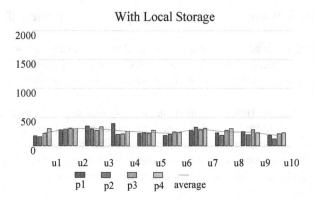

Fig. 4. Posture design: time using local storage

The second parameter we measured with time is the time the system takes to update the skeleton in the virtual editor (Fig. 1-C) and in the posture list. The average time without using local storage was 758 ms. When using local storage the average time was 152 ms.

Regarding user's satisfaction, the SUS satisfaction questionnaire was used [1]. In this test, users express their agreement with 10 sentences after performing the task. For each sentence, a score between 1 and 5 is given, meaning 1 strongly disagreement and 5 strongly agreement. Then, based on these values, the SUS satisfaction questionnaire final value is calculated. This value can be between 0 and 100. A final value near 100 indicates complete satisfaction.

The final result for the SUS test for users that performed the task without using local storage was 72.5, indicating that users were almost satisfied with the system. The final result for the SUS test for users that performed the task using local storage was 86, indicating that users were satisfied with the system.

5   Discussion

We made the improvement of using local storage in the system tailored by the idea of reducing response time within the application. The evaluation shows results that support the expected improvement as well of other improvement: the enhancement of the usability in the system.

The first and more visible result is the reduction of the time when performing tasks (as shown in Figs. 2 and 3). In overall, in posture design the average time decreased in more than 1 s when using local storage from 1398 ms to 252 ms. Regarding the time to update the skeleton in the virtual editor there was a reduction in average of 506 ms. These improvements make the application easiest to use and makes the user feels more comfortable and secure using it. That is because the actions he or she is performing are reflected almost immediately within the virtual environment.

But the most important finding within the evaluation is the improvement of the usability in the system. The SUS test shows us the aspects where the application improves using local storage. A deep analysis of the scores associated with the SUS test sentences (depicted in Table 1) reveals some important aspects. Only the sentences 3, 6, 7, 8 and 9 have different scores. In the case of the sentence 3, users think the system using local storage is easiest to use. For the sentence 6, users without using local storage say that there was too much inconsistency. In sentence 7 users think that the system using local storage is fastest to learn to use. But the bigger differences are in sentences 8 and 9 (more than one point). That indicates, in the case of sentence 8, that users think the system without local storage is a bit cumbersome to use. Finally, according the sentence 9, users totally agree that they felt very confident using the system when using local storage. All users give 5 out of 5 points to this sentence. That's not the case when they are using the system without local storage. In this case, the sentence is scored with 3,8.

Table 1. SUS score for each sentence within the evaluation

SUS sentence	Score	
	Without	With
1 - I think that I would like to use this system frequently	3,8	3,8
2 - I found the system unnecessarily complex	1,6	1,6
3 - I thought the system was easy to use	4	4,8
4 - I think that I would need the support of a technical person to be able to use this system	1,8	1,8
5 - I found the various functions in this system were well integrated	3,8	3,8
6 - I thought there was too much inconsistency in this system	2,4	1,4
7 - I would imagine that most people would learn to use this system very quickly	3,6	4,6
8 - I found the system very cumbersome to use	2,6	1,2
9 - I felt very confident using the system	3,8	5
10 - I needed to learn a lot of things before I could get going with this system	1,6	1,6

The results of the test confirm how the improvement of the system solves the problems found in the performance and presentation translations within the interaction process (Fig. 2). Now, the interaction cycle reflects the outputs according the users' inputs in a way the user feels totally confortable. As a result, the usability of the system improves, as reflected in the SUS score.

6   Conclusions and Future Work

In this paper we presented an improvement for the posture design process in a rehabilitation system. We found the weaknesses within the interactive process that make less usable the system. Then, we discussed how web technologies, such as local storage and offline Web applications can improve user interaction with the system. As a result, we introduced locally information management in the local client. To that end, we use local storage present in all major browsers.

To measure the improvement in the usability of the system we perform an evaluation. The evaluation shows that with the use of local storage the interactive cycle was improved, solving the problems found in some of the translations of the interactive process. Also, the usability of the system was improved, as reflected by the SUS test, and users felt more confident using the system.

As a future work we'll continue the improvement of the system using web technologies to improve user satisfaction in rehabilitation applications.

Acknowledgments. This work has been partially supported by project TSI-100101-2013-147 from the Spanish Ministry of Industry, Energy and Tourism and the fellowship 2014/10340 from the University of Castilla-La Mancha.

References

1. Abowd, G.D.: Formal aspects of human-computer interaction. Ph.D. thesis (1991)
2. Marco, F.A., Gallud, J., Penichet, V.M.R., Winckler, M.: A model-based approach for supporting offline interaction with web sites resilient to interruptions. In: Sheng, Q.Z., Kjeldskov, J. (eds.) ICWE 2013. LNCS, vol. 8295, pp. 156–171. Springer, Cham (2013). doi: 10.1007/978-3-319-04244-2_15
3. Albertos Marco, F., Fernández Valls, J.A., Penichet, V.M.R., Lozano, M.D., Gallud, J.A.: Improving postures design in virtual rehabilitation environments. In: Fardoun, H.M., Gamito, P., Penichet, V.M.R., Alghazzawi, D.M. (eds.) Proceedings of the 3rd 2015 Workshop on ICTs for improving Patients Rehabilitation Research Techniques (REHAB 2015), pp. 89–92. ACM, New York (2015). http://dx.doi.org/10.1145/2838944.2838966
4. Brooke, J.: SUS - a quick and dirty usability scale. In: Usability Evaluation in Industry (1996)
5. Constantinescu, L., Pradana, R., Kim, J., Gong, P., Fulham, M., Feng, D.: Rich internet application system for patient-centric healthcare data management using handheld devices. In: Annual International Conference of the IEEE Engineering in Medicine and Biology Society. EMBC 2009. pp. 5167, 5170, 3–6 September 2009 (2009). http://dx.doi.org/10.1109/IEMBS.2009.5332734
6. Ferriol, M.P., Alcalde, V.M.A., Tous, X., Meliá, M., Sastre, T.J., Farrency, B.M.A., Ponce, M.E., Llano, P.B., Mas, S.R.: Play for Health 2.0: Evolving P4H to a Web Environment Using HTML5 and JavaScript. In VI International Conference on eHealth, Telemedicine, and Social Medicine (eTELEMED), IARIA Barcelona, Spain, ISSN: 2308-4359. pp. 44–78. ISBN: 978-1-61208-327-8 (2014)
7. Garrido, J.E., Marset, I., Penichet, V.M., Lozano, M.D.: Balance disorder rehabilitation through movement interaction. In: Proceedings of the 7th International Conference on Pervasive Computing Technologies for Healthcare (PervasiveHealth 2013). ICST (Institute for Computer Sciences, Social-Informatics and Telecommunications Engineering), ICST, Brussels, Belgium, Belgium, pp. 319–322 (2013). http://dx.doi.org/10.4108/icst.pervasivehealth.2013.252368
8. Kayama, H., Nishiguchi, S., Yamada, M., Aoyama, T., Okamoto, K., Kuroda, T.: Effect of a Kinect-based exercise game on improving executive cognitive performance in community-dwelling elderly. In: Proceedings of the 7th International Conference on Pervasive Computing Technologies for Healthcare (PervasiveHealth 2013). ICST (Institute for Computer Sciences, Social-Informatics and Telecommunications Engineering), ICST, Brussels, Belgium, Belgium, pp. 362–365 (2013). http://dx.doi.org/10.4108/icst.pervasivehealth.2013.252253

9. Lange, B., Koenig, S., McConnell, E., Chang, C.-Y., Juang, R., Suma, E., Bolas, M., Rizzo, A.: Interactive game-based rehabilitation using the Microsoft Kinect. In: Proceedings of the 2012 IEEE Virtual Reality (VR 2012), pp. 171–172. IEEE Computer Society, Washington, DC (2012). http://dx.doi.org/10.1109/VR.2012.6180935

10. Lozano-Quilis, J.A., Gil-Gómez, H., Gil-Gómez, J.A., Albiol-Pérez, S., Palacios, G., Fardoum, H.M., Mashat, A.S.: Virtual reality system for multiple sclerosis rehabilitation using KINECT. In: Proceedings of the 7th International Conference on Pervasive Computing Technologies for Healthcare (PervasiveHealth 2013). ICST (Institute for Computer Sciences, Social-Informatics and Telecommunications Engineering), ICST, Brussels, Belgium, Belgium, pp. 366–369 (2013). http://dx.doi.org/10.4108/icst.pervasivehealth.2013.252208

11. McAllister, P., Bond, R.: An offline web app for the self-management of diabetes and obesity. In: 2014 Irish Human Computer Interaction Conference. Dublin (2014). http://ihci2014.dcu.ie/style/papers/Full/Patrick McAllister and Raymond Bond_An Offline Web App for the Self-Management of Diabetes and Obesity.pdf

12. POSEFY: http://www.posefy.com/. Accessed Jul 2015

13. Putnam, C., Cheng, J., Rusch, D., Berthiaume, A., Burke, R.: Supporting therapists in motion-based gaming for brain injury rehabilitation. In: CHI 2013 Extended Abstracts on Human Factors in Computing Systems (CHI EA 2013), pp. 391–396. ACM, New York (2013). http://doi.acm.org/10.1145/2468356.2468426

14. Tous, F., et al.: Play for health: videogame platform for motor and cognitive telerehabilitation of patients. In: The Third International Conference on eHealth, Telemedicine and Social Medicine (eTELEMED 2011), IARIA, February 2011, pp. 59–63

15. W3C: Offline Web Applications (2008). http://www.w3.org/TR/offline-webapps/

16. W3C: Web Database (2010). http://www.w3.org/TR/webdatabase/

17. W3C: HTML5 A vocabulary and associated APIs for HTML and XHTML. W3C Recommendation 28 October 2014. http://www.w3.org/TR/html5/. Accessed Jun 2015

18. W3C: Indexed Database API (2015). http://www.w3.org/TR/IndexedDB/

19. W3C: Web Storage. Editor's Draft 14 May 2014. http://dev.w3.org/html5/webstorage. Accessed Jun 2015

20. W3C: File API: Directories and System (2016). https://www.w3.org/TR/file-system-api/

21. W3C: Service Workers (2015). https://slightlyoff.github.io/ServiceWorker/spec/service_worker/

22. WebExercises: http://www.webexercises.com/. Accessed Jul 2015

A Stationary Bike in Augmented Audio Reality. An Investigation on Soundscapes Influence on Preferred Biking Speed

Justyna Maculewicz[✉] and Stefania Serafin

M-LAB, Aalborg University Copenhagen, Copenhagen, Denmark
{jma,sts}@create.aau.dk

Abstract. In this article we present the results of an experiment where participants were asked to bike with selected soundscapes to measure their preferred pace and perception of the several aspects of the soundscapes. The results show that indeed different soundscapes can manipulate preferred pace of a biking person. This experiment is the first step into designing a system for rhythmic rehabilitation based on a stationary bike augmented in an audio reality. A concept of the system is as well presented. The specific sensors will be used to monitor users' pace and heart rate while exercising and manipulate audio feedback and cues. Simple technology solutions will allow for the system to be used by the wide range of users. The innovation is to use as a feedback and cues ecological sounds, which has power to manipulate a bikers' pace and give a more natural experience.

Keywords: Stationary bike · Rehabilitation · Soundscape · Audio augmented reality

1 Introduction

Music is very often used for motivation and exercise entrainment. It serves as a pace's cue in rhythmic rehabilitation. Properly adjusted music tempo, which fits user's preferences helps exercise longer with higher satisfaction. Already developed systems allow for usage of user's pulse for estimating correct music tempo specifically adjusted to users needs.

We are developing a simple system centred on a stationary bike, where magnet sensor placed on the one side of a bike and magnet placed on a pedal is responsible for detecting rounds per minute (RPM) performed by the user. Before, we tested it with a simple drum signal [10], but our ultimate goal is to use ecological signals for indicating speed of the person.

This article is an extension of the original work published in ACM [9].

1.1 A Concept of an Exercising System

As it was done in the running application systems [7,12], we want to incorporate as well heart rate sensor as a tool for matching background sounds with

© Springer International Publishing AG 2017
H.M. Fardoun et al. (Eds.): REHAB 2015, CCIS 665, pp. 162–178, 2017.
https://doi.org/10.1007/978-3-319-69694-2_15

the users' performance. From our research in interactive walking area [8], we know that soundscape sounds can influence humans walking pace. We believe that the same effect will be achieved if we introduce soundscape sounds in biking. Both, auditory feedback and soundscape sounds will be controlled through users' performance, which will give them a sense of immersion into the auditory reality, help to control their performance and match stimulation with expected fatigue. Music gives indication of a tempo, which user should match. We want to introduce a system, which is more flexible and do not force users to bike in a certain pace, but give them impression of relative speed, which in they should bike. By measuring heart rate we can see if the person is biking too fast or too slow to achieve the expected results. The system will manipulate the soundscape sounds based on the programmed rules and information gained from the user at the beginning of the session. The system is meant for the everyday users of the stationary bikes, who are not able to exercise outside or it is too difficult or dangerous for them. It is not a system for professional bikers, who should achieve specific, high goals during training. By introducing soundscapes into trainings we want to give users higher satisfaction from training, divert their attention from fatigue and give a cue and motivation for the relative changes in pace while training. Since no rhythmic sounds will be incorporated into soundscapes, pace of the user can be easily adjusted and a level of frustration lowered since the goal is not to achieve specific tempo but a relative to the level of the performed one. Ecological feedback, which will be introduced based on the information from magnet sensors will help to monitor performance for the user. He or she can have an idea of their tempo stability, speed and acceleration. These sounds will simulate ground on which person imagines to bike and it will fit soundscape sounds.

1.2   Soundscape

The term soundscape was introduced by R. Murray Schafer in 1960s and the research on this topic was pioneered by The World Soundscape Project (WSP) - an educational and research group established by R. Murray Schafer at Simon Fraser University. Soundscapes mediate the relations between environment and people who perceive them. According to The International Organization for Standardization (ISO) a soundscape is a perceptual construct, related to but distinguished from a physical phenomenon (acoustic environment) (ISO 12913-1:2014). As a working theory used in The Positive Soundscape Project [4] states, soundscape is "the totality of all sounds within a location with an emphasis on the relationship between individual's or society's perception of, understanding of and interaction with the sonic environment". Soundscapes exist through human perception of the acoustic environment. Humans' assessment of the soundscapes is driven by high-level cognitive features rather than low-level acoustic characteristics [4]. The perception of what is positive or negative soundscape is driven by the meaning and emotion carried by the soundscape sounds. People prefer the soundscapes where the natural sounds and human sounds are incorporated [4,5]. Further results of The Positive Soundscape Project indicated participants' need of having behavioural and cognitive control over it. Soundscape sounds should carry information and be not persistent. Those which require more attention are being assessed as negative. Sounds, which 'blend together', are assessed as positive. Research on combined landscape and soundscape done by Brambilla [2] showed that the level of evoked annoyance is lower and its acceptability higher when a sound is more congruent with the listener's expectations.

Until this time we did not find any research which assess human rhythmic behaviour when exposed to the various soundscapes. We can derive some general assumption from the Boltz's [1] study. Her results showed that people tend to speed up their preferred tempo when exposed to annoying sounds and slow down when exposed to relaxing music. Franěk [6] observed rhythmic behaviour of their subjects when walking in natural environment. He concluded that people walk faster in places without greenery and with a higher level of traffic and noise in places with greenery and with a low level of traffic and noise.

The first step in a process of designing the above mention system is to evaluate if soundscapes have indeed power to manipulate preferred pace of a biker. Firstly, in the article we describe more precisely the stages of the system development and further we investigate experimentally if the chosen soundscapes motivate our participants to bike in different pace.

2 The System

2.1 The Basic Idea

We are introducing a rehabilitation and exercising system, which is based on the idea of a potential pace change by modifying soundscape sounds. Information from the user about their expected results from a training, actual pace and heart rate will influence feedback and soundscape sounds presented while training. A soundscape's selection will be based on our previous research [8] and preferences of the users. We will start from introducing a few examples and develop with the first volunteers, who will agree to test our system. In the final implementation, a selection of soundscapes will be broad but finite. Figure 1 presents a visualisation of the concept.

Sensors Application. First, user chooses their goal (e.g. challenge, relax), initial soundscape and feedback sounds. While riding, the system will take into account information collected from the user at the beginning of the session, heart rate and pedaling rate. Pedaling rate will control feedback and heart rate will control soundscape which change should motivate user to accelerate, decelerate or stay at the same level of pedaling rate.

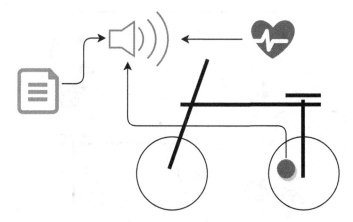

Fig. 1. A visualisation of the basic idea standing behind the system. Information collected from the users, heart rate sensor and magnet sensor will influence feedback and soundscape sounds presented to the users.

2.2   Research Phase

The initial tests will be performed in the university lab facilities. Magnet sensor will be connected to microcontroller Arduino and data transported to the computer where engine system will run. The core of the software will be Max/MSP from cycling74 where on-line sound modeling will be performed based on the predefined assumptions and users input. Figure 2 presents a visualisation of the initial implementation.

2.3   The Final Implementation

Based on the results of the research and after usefulness and efficiency of the system will be confirmed, we are planning to implement it as a smart phone application. Figure 3 presents a visualisation of the final implementation.

3   Experimental Investigations

The below described experiment is the first stage of experimental investigation towards augmented rehabilitation system. The goal was to check if different soundscapes can manipulate a bikers' preferred tempo while using a stationary bike. As well, we asked our participants to judge several aspects of the soundscapes to search for the possible explanation of the expected tempo manipulation. Based on the internal clock theory [13] we assume that more arousing soundscape will motivate to faster biking. As well, we hypothesise that soundscape perceived as faster in listening tests, will motivate to faster biking.

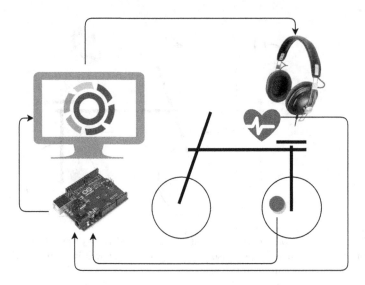

Fig. 2. A visualisation of the initial implementation. Data collected by heart rate and magnet sensors will be collected and transferred by microcontroller Arduino to the computer, where our implementation developed in Max/MSP software will calculate predicted changes and synthesis sounds to be presented to the users.

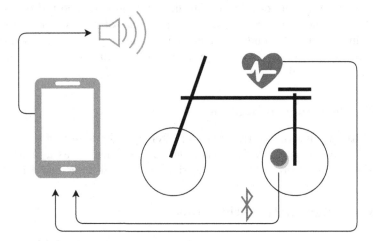

Fig. 3. A visualisation of the final implementation that is based on a smart phone application and Bluetooth communication between sensors and main software.

3.1 Participants and Procedure

A total of 16 participants (8 males, 8 females), aged between 19–40 years (M = 35.8 years, SD = 7.8), took part in the experiment. All participants reported having normal or corrected-to-normal hearing. No compensation was offered for participation.

The participants performed a total of 4 listening trials and 4 biking trials in randomised order within each sub-experiment. During each listening trial participants were asked to listen to the soundscapes for 30 s each and answer several questions concerning their perception of the soundscapes. During each biking trial, participants were asked to bike in their preferred tempo on a stationary bike and as well answer several questions concerning their biking experience with each soundscape.

3.2 Setup and Stimuli

We chose 4 different soundscapes to be tested in the experiment. The choice was driven by the results of our previous experiment [8] and personal preferences. Our previous experiment showed that soundscapes such us 'seashore' and 'busy street' can significantly manipulate preferred walking pace. We decided to use them as well in the present experiment. Two additional soundscapes were chosen to supplement the experimental design. Particularly, we chose 'delicate rainy forest' and 'storm with quite street noise in the background'. The stimuli intensity was adjusted to the comfortable level. The mean power measured by PRAAT software was: seashore – 63.1 dB, forest – 72.3 dB, street – 72.53 dB, and storm 72.8 dB. The participants were allowed to adjust the volume level if it was not comfortable, but at the end, non of them decided to do so.

During the listening task, participants were asked to seat on a chair and listen to each soundscape for 30 s. We used Sennheiser HD 600 headphones and Fireface 800 sound card for soundscapes playback. The questionnaire was presented on paper and participants wrote their answers on an answer card. During the biking task, participants used a regular stationary bike and the same playback system. The questionnaire was presented on paper in front of them. This time, to make the procedure more comfortable (participants could stayed on a bike), participants were giving their answer verbally and a researcher wrote them down on a dedicated answer card.

3.3 Measures

A combination of behavioural and self-reported measures were used to gather data during the experiment.

The participants' personal opinion on the soundscapes was administrated by the utilisation of the questionnaire:

Ql1 To which extend you perceive this soundscape as pleasant? ('1' = very pleasant, '7' = very unpleasant).

Ql2 How do you perceive presented soundscape? ('1' = very calming, '7' = very arousing).

Ql3 How do you perceive tempo of this soundscape? ('1' = very slow, '7' = very fast).

Ql4 How do you perceive valence of the presented soundscape? ('1' = very positive, '7' = very negative).

In regards to the participants' behaviour, their biking RPM (rounds per minute) was logged in order to provide an estimate of their preferred tempo. Particularly, whenever a participant passed a magnet sensor placed on a side of a bike, tempo of a one round of pedalling was logged.

The participants' experience of each condition was assessed by means of a questionnaire administered after each trial.

Qb1 How difficult it was to bike while listening to the soundscape? ('1' = very difficult, '7' = very easy).

Qb2 The pace I kept while biking was: ('1' = very slow, '7' = very fast).

Qb3 Biking with this soundscape felt natural: ('1' = completely agree, '7' = completely disagree).

Qb4 I felt comfortable while biking with this soundscape: ('1' = completely agree, '7' = completely disagree).

Qb5 I would like to listen to this soundscape while biking: ('1' = completely agree, '7' = completely disagree).

3.4   Results

We performed analysis using One-way Repeated Measure ANOVA for metric data and Friedman's ANOVA and Wilcoxon test for ordinal data. The choice of these tests was driven by the experiment design (one independent variable with four levels and within-subjects design). Additionally we performed Spearmann correlation for comparison of all of obtained data (RPM and Ql1–Qb5).

Listening Test: Questionnaire. Table 1 shows the results of Friedman's ANOVA performed on the answers for Ql1–Ql4. We can see that for each question was revealed significant difference between soundscapes (Table 1). Figures 4, 5, 6 and 7 present visualisation of the results for each question. Wilcoxon test revealed significant differences within all of the stimuli pairwise comparisons within each question. We can see general pattern that seashore sound was perceived as the most pleasant, the slowest, the most calming, and the most positive. On the other hand street soundscape was perceived as the most unpleasant, the most arousing, the fastest, and the most negative. Forest and storm soundscapes are in between with general lower values for the forest soundscape.

In general, the street soundscape has always been placed on the opposite part of the scale than the other soundscapes. As the only one, it was perceived on average as unpleasant, arousing, fast and negative. A few participants rated similarly the storm soundscapes, but the median rating for storm was always below 4.

Biking: Preferred Pace. One-way repeated measure ANOVA revealed significant difference between RPM rate when biking with different soundscapes $F(3, 45) = 5.52$, $p < 0.05$. The Bonferroni post hoc test showed differences between specific soundscapes obtained during analysis. Table 2 and Fig. 8 present these differences. Figure 9 visualise the results of the average RPM for each participant.

Table 1. Summary of the results of Friedman's ANOVA test for the questionnaire data obtained in the listening test.

Questions	χ^2	p
Ql1	43.78	<0.001
Ql2	37.48	<0.001
Ql3	41.66	<0.001
Ql4	34.19	<0.001

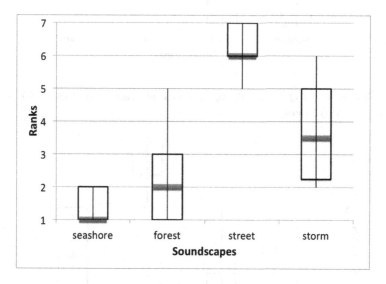

Fig. 4. The results of Ql1: To which extend you perceive this soundscape as pleasant? ('1' = very pleasant, '7' = very unpleasant).

Table 2. Summary of the significant differences between specified soundscapes (Bonferroni post-hoc test) for the RPM variable.

Soundscapes	Mean diff.	Std. dev.	p
Seashore vs forest	−4.29	2.63	0.79
Seashore vs street	−9.8	2.15	<0.05
Seashore vs storm	−7.28	2.31	<0.05
Forest vs street	−5.61	2.26	0.15
Forest vs storm	−3.1	2.84	1.00
Street vs storm	2.51	2.94	1.00

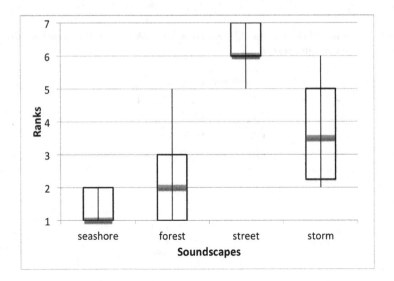

Fig. 5. The results of Ql2: How do you perceive presented soundscape? ('1' = very calming, '7' = very arousing).

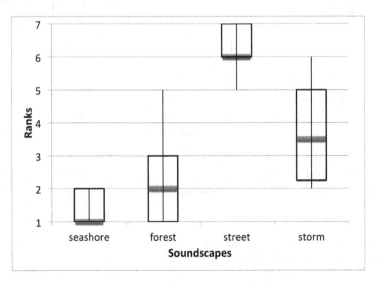

Fig. 6. The results of Ql3: How do you perceive tempo of this soundscape? ('1' = very slow, '7' = very fast).

Biking: Questionnaire. Table 3 presents the results of Friedman's ANOVA performed on the answers for biking questionnaire. It can be observed that soundscapes differentiated significantly answers for Qb2, Qb4, and Qb5. Figures 10, 11, 12, 13 and 14 visualise the answers for each question subsequently. We can see that questions Qb1 and Qb3 did not differentiate significantly the average

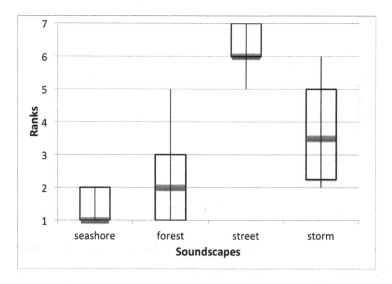

Fig. 7. The results of Ql4: How do you perceive valence of the presented soundscape? ('1' = very positive, '7' = very negative).

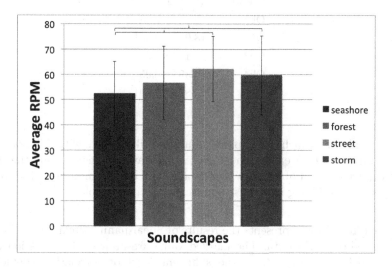

Fig. 8. The average RPM rate for each soundscape. The horizontal brackets indicate significant differences ($p < 0.05$)

rating of the soundscapes. Participants reported that the ease of biking and naturalness of this experience was quite similar for all of the tested variables. On the other hand, the perceived speed and comfort of biking significantly differentiated the ratings of the soundscapes. Participants as well, to significantly different extent would like to listen to the soundscapes while biking. Although, only the street soundscape was rated on average above 4, which means that this

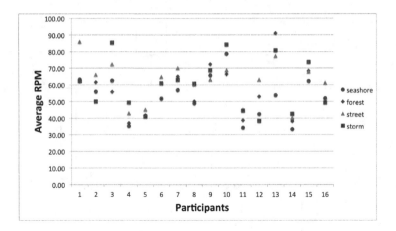

Fig. 9. The average RPM rate for each soundscape and each participant.

Table 3. Summary of the results of Friedman's ANOVA test for the questionnaire data obtained in the biking test.

Questions	χ^2	p
Qb1	3.81	=0.28
Qb2	18.02	<0.001
Qb3	3.17	=0.37
Qb4	10.39	<0.05
Qb5	23.86	<0.001

one is the only one which participants would not like to bike with. The rating of comfort varies a lot for each soundscapes, but on average, again, only the street soundscape was rated above 4, which means that participants did not perceive the experience of biking with this soundscape as comfortable.

Correlations. Table 4 presents the results of Spearmann correlation performed on all of the obtained data. The marked value are above 0.6 correlation coefficient, which we accepted, as the sufficient level of correlation coefficient. Although, we are aware, that good practise suggest to take into account only those above 0.8. We treat this study as exploratory. Higher rigorous will be applied in the future studies with the soundscapes designed with higher level of control, based on the initial guidelines emerging from this study and literature.

3.5   Discussion of the Experiment Results

With this experiment we aimed to show the influence of different types of soundscape on preferred biking pace measured in RPMs. With the questionnaires we aimed to analyse the perceived characteristics of the chosen soundscapes.

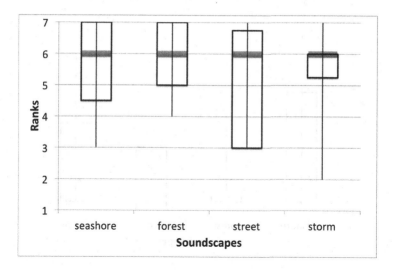

Fig. 10. The results of Qb1: How difficult it was to bike while listening to the sound-scape? ('1' = very difficult, '7' = very easy).

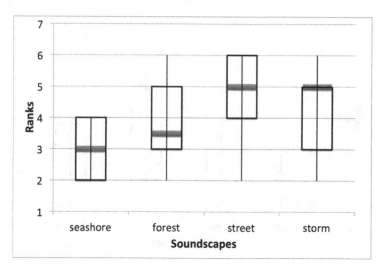

Fig. 11. The results of Qb2: The pace I kept while biking was: ('1' = very slow, '7' = very fast).

We hoped to find significant correlation between several measures to be able to explain the reasons standing behind manipulated pace. We can definitely conclude that soundscapes sounds have power to significantly manipulate preferred biking tempo, however, there is high variability between participants. As we expected, participants were biking on average the slowest with seashore sound-scape and the fastest with street soundscape.

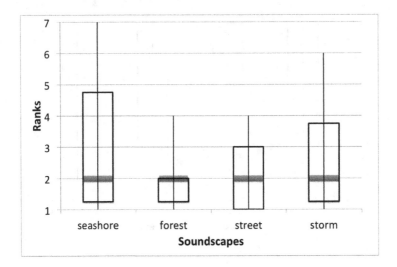

Fig. 12. The results of Qb3: Biking with this soundscape felt natural: ('1' = completely agree, '7' = completely disagree).

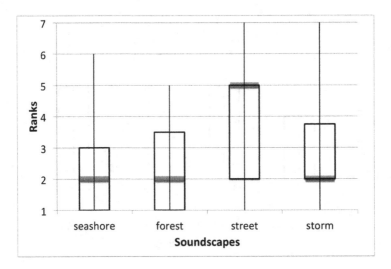

Fig. 13. The results of Qb4: I felt comfortable while biking with this soundscape: ('1' = completely agree, '7' = completely disagree).

The effect of changing tempo while biking with different soundscapes can be explained from the two different perspectives, the entrainment theory and the internal clock theory. The first perspective suggests that humans perceive and synchronise with environmental rhythms in a three-stages process. First, the rhythmic signal needs to be detected, than the rhythmic signal has to be produced by a person and the last one is integration of sensory information and

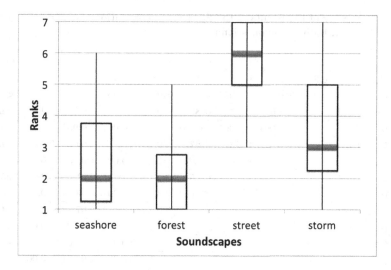

Fig. 14. The results of Qb5: I would like to listen to this soundscape while biking: ('1' = completely agree, '7' = completely disagree).

motor production [11]. We did not mean to apply any rhythmic components to the soundscapes, but participants could get the general feeling of the speed of the soundscape, through the recurring elements (e.g. waves in the seashore sound-scape, or cars in street soundscape) or the general amount amount of events happening within specified length of time. We can see on Figs. 6 and 8 that the pattern of differences between soundscape and average tempo and rating of per-ceived tempo are similar, but when we check the correlation between tempo and ratings of Ql3 Table 4 it can be seen that the correlation coefficient is pretty low (0.39), however the correlation is significant ($p < 0.05$). The second perspective, which could be used to explain the effect comes from the internal clock theory [13]. As many authors mention increased arousal affects the internal clock rate (e.g. [1,3]). Again, the pattern of differences between ratings for arousal and average tempo is similar. The participants rated street soundscape as the most arousing and and seashore as the most calming. However, correlation coefficient between these two measures is pretty low (0.36), but the correlation is significant ($p < 0.05$). We conclude that the perceived speed and calming – arousal rating can only partially explain the differences in average RPM rates.

Since soundscapes are analysed at the higher cognitive levels, we believe that information and memories stored in the soundscapes can influence the preferred tempo. In general seashore and forest soundscapes are associated with relaxing moments where people tend to live in slower pace. On the other hand street and storm soundscapes are associated with faster actions. Street contained the biggest amount of machine-like sounds and seashore and forest – nature sounds. Storm was a combination of the nature sounds with very quiet traffic noise.

Table 4. Summary of the results of the Spearmann correlation test performed on the average RPM and both of the questionnaires.

Variable		Ql1	Ql2	Ql3	Ql4	Qb1	Qb2	Qb3	Qb4	Qb5
RPM	Corr. coeff.	0.2	0.36	0.39	0.25	0.01	**0.65**	0.11	0.33	0.36
	p	=0.12	<0.05	<0.05	<0.05	=0.94	<0.001	=0.4	<0.05	<0.05
Ql1	Corr. coeff.		**0.85**	**0.77**	**0.89**	−0.18	0.45	−0.0	0.42	**0.63**
	p		<0.001	<0.001	<0.001	=0.15	<0.001	=0.98	=0.001	<0.001
Ql2	Corr. coeff.			**0.82**	**0.87**	−0.15	0.56	0.04	0.43	**0.64**
	p			<0.001	<0.001	=0.24	<0.001	=0.98	<0.001	<0.001
Ql3	Corr. coeff.				**0.75**	−0.13	0.48	0.01	0.34	0.5
	p				<0.001	0.32	<0.001	0.96	<0.05	<0.001
Ql4	Corr. coeff.					−0.25	0.48	0.07	0.52	**0.67**
	p					<0.05	<0.001	=0.59	<0.001	<0.001
Qb1	Corr. coeff.						0.0	**-0.61**	−0.59	−0.35
	p						=0.99	<0.001	<0.001	<0.05
Qb2	Corr. coeff.							−0.01	0.37	0.42
	p							=0.93	<0.05	=0.001
Qb3	Corr. coeff.								**0.64**	0.39
	p								<0.001	=0.001
Qb4	Corr. coeff.									**0.75**
	p									<0.001

The correlation coefficient for RPM values and questionnaire ratings got sufficiently high (>0.6) only when correlated with the answers for Qb2, which means that participants were decently aware of the changing pace. In general, all of the answers for the questionnaire presented in listening data correlated with each other. We can see that more pleasant soundscape was as well perceived as more calming, slow, and positive. These measures correlated, except the perceived speed, at a sufficient level with the willingness of listening to the soundscape while biking. The questionnaire presented during biking trials revealed interesting correlation between Qb1 and Qb3. The more soundscape was perceived as difficult the less natural it was. As well, the level of perceived naturalness correlated on a sufficient level with the feeling of comfort and willingness to bike with the soundscape.

4   Conclusions

In this paper we presented a simple system for exercise and rehabilitation, which especially could be used by elderly who are not able to train outside or feel afraid of going out alone. A core of the system is a stationary bike with incorporated sensors for controlling pedalling and heart rate. The goal is to motivate users to bike in a pace, which is faster or slower from their preferred one. It is to challenge them but also control their fatigue and motivate them to slow down if they bike to fast and their heart rate is too high. We see the final implementation as a smart phone application with broad but selected soundscapes and feedback sounds.

Based on the experimental investigations we can definitely conclude that soundscape sounds can influence the average preferred pace of a biker while using a stationary bike. There are several characteristics of the soundscapes, which we tested while looking for explanation of this effect. We can conclude only on partial effects which the arousal, valence, pleasantness, and perceived speed can have on the preferred tempo. There is a need for more complex experiment design when the soundscape will be designed with specific parameters in mind such us: the amount of human, nature, and machine-like sounds; the general amount of events which will not be perceived as background (e.g. cars, birds, thunders). Since we operate mostly on questionnaire data, which are ordinal, we should perform the future experiments on a bigger group of people. The analysis of correlation between questionnaire items shows that people would like to listen to soundscapes while biking which pleasant, calming, positive, and comfortable. The naturalness, perceived speed, and difficulty were not that important.

References

1. Boltz, M.G.: Changes in internal tempo and effects on the learning and remembering of event durations. J. Exp. Psychol. Learn. Memory Cogn. **20**(5), 1154 (1994)
2. Brambilla, G., Maffei, L.: Responses to noise in urban parks and in rural quiet areas. Acta Acustica united with Acustica **92**(6), 881–886 (2006)
3. Burle, B., Casini, L.: Dissociation between activation and attention effects in time estimation: implications for internal clock models. J. Exp. Psychol. Hum. Percept. Perform. **27**(1), 195 (2001)
4. Davies, W.J., Adams, M.D., Bruce, N.S., Cain, R., Carlyle, A., Cusack, P., Hall, D.A., Hume, K.I., Irwin, A., Jennings, P., et al.: Perception of soundscapes: an interdisciplinary approach. Appl. Acoust. **74**(2), 224–231 (2013)
5. Dubois, D., Guastavino, C., Raimbault, M.: A cognitive approach to urban soundscapes: Using verbal data to access everyday life auditory categories. Acta acustica united with acustica **92**(6), 865–874 (2006)
6. Franěk, M.: Environmental factors influencing pedestrian walking speed. Percept. Motor Skills **116**(3), 992–1019 (2013)
7. Hockman, J.A., Wanderley, M.M., Fujinaga, I.: Real-time phase vocoder manipulation by runners pace. In: Proceedings of the International Conference on New Interfaces for Musical Expression, pp. 90–93. Citeseer (2009)
8. Maculewicz, J., Erkut, C., Serafin, S.: An investigation on the influence of soundscapes and footstep sounds in affecting preferred walking pace. In: Proceedings of the 21st International Conference on Auditory Display (ICAD 2015) (2015)
9. Maculewicz, J., Serafin, S.: A stationary bike in augmented audio reality. In: Proceedings of the 3rd 2015 Workshop on ICTs for Improving Patients Rehabilitation Research Techniques, pp. 164–166. ACM (2015)
10. Maculewicz, J., Serafin, S., Kofoed, L.B.: Following tempo on an exercising bike with and without auditory feedback. In: CMMR 2013, pp. 834–843 (2013)
11. Phillips-Silver, J., Aktipis, C.A., Bryant, G.A.: The ecology of entrainment: foundations of coordinated rhythmic movement. Music Percept. **28**(1), 3 (2010)

12. Rubisch, J., Husinsky, M., Doppler, J., Raffaseder, H., Horsak, B., Ambichl, B., Figl, A.: A mobile music concept as support for achieving target heart rate in preventive and recreational endurance training. In: Proceedings of the 5th Audio Mostly Conference: A Conference on Interaction with Sound, p. 19. ACM (2010)
13. Treisman, M.: Temporal discrimination and the indifference interval: implications for a model of the "internal clock". Psychol. Monogr. Gen. Appl. **77**(13), 1 (1963)

Author Index

Abou-Tair, Dhiah el Diehn I.   126
Alazrai, Rami   126
Albertos-Marco, Félix   150
Alghazzawi, Daniyal M.   94
Alhusseini, Abdullah   126
Alhwayan, Ekhlass   126
Almeida, T.   69

Bento, Bruno   141
Blasco, Sonia   59, 83
Bonfanti, Silvia   116
Brito, R.   69
Brito, Rodrigo   141
Buzzi, Maria Claudia   1
Buzzi, Marina   1

Caçoête, C.   69
Cano, Sandra   94
Carboni, Andrea   46
Chirivella, Javier   59, 83
Collazos, César   94
Comotti, Claudio   35
Curzio, Olivia   46

Daoud, Mohammad I.   126

Fardoun, Habib M.   94
Fernández Valls, José Antonio   150

Gagliardo, Pablo   59, 83
Gallud, José A.   150
Gameiro, Fátima   141
Gamito, P.   69
Gamito, Pedro   26, 141
Gargantini, Angelo   116

Iacoviello, Daniela   12

Leandro, A.   69
Lopes, P.   69
Lopes, Paulo   141
Lozano, María Dolores   150
Lv, Zhihan   59, 83, 106

Maculewicz, Justyna   162
Magrini, Massimo   46
Morais, D.   69
Morais, Diogo   26, 141

Neto, Margarida   141

Oliveira, H.   69
Oliveira, J.   69
Oliveira, Jorge   26, 141

Pavlovic, Matthew   26
Penades, Vicente   59, 83
Peñeñory, Victor   94
Penichet, Víctor M.R.   150
Petracca, Andrea   12
Placidi, Giuseppe   12

Qadoummi, Talal   126

Regazzoni, Daniele   35
Rizzi, Caterina   35
Rosa, B.   69
Rosa, Pedro J.   26

Salvetti, Ovidio   46
Serafin, Stefania   162
Shihan, Dima   126
Smyth, Olivia   26
Spezialetti, Matteo   12

Trujillo, Amaury   1

Vitali, Andrea   35

Printed in the United States
By Bookmasters